Emerging Biomaterials and Techniques in Tissue Regeneration

Editor

ALAN S. HERFORD

ORAL AND MAXILLOFACIAL SURGERY CLINICS OF NORTH AMERICA

www.oralmaxsurgery.theclinics.com

Consulting Editor
RICHARD H. HAUG

February 2017 • Volume 29 • Number 1

ELSEVIER

1600 John F. Kennedy Boulevard • Suite 1800 • Philadelphia, Pennsylvania, 19103-2899

http://www.oralmaxsurgery.theclinics.com

ORAL AND MAXILLOFACIAL SURGERY CLINICS OF NORTH AMERICA Volume 29, Number 1
February 2017 ISSN 1042-3699, ISBN-13: 978-0-323-49667-4

Editor: John Vassallo; j.vassallo@elsevier.com
Developmental Editor: Colleen Dietzler

Oral and Maxillofacial Surgery Clinics of North America (ISSN 1042-3699) is published quarterly by Elsevier Inc., 360 Park Avenue South, New York, NY 10010-1710. Months of issue are February, May, August, and November. Business and Editorial Offices: 1600 John F. Kennedy Blvd., Suite 1800, Philadelphia, PA 19103-2899. Periodicals postage paid at New York, NY and additional mailing offices. Subscription prices are $385.00 per year for US individuals, $653.00 per year for US institutions, $100.00 per year for US students and residents, $455.00 per year for Canadian individuals, $783.00 per year for Canadian institutions, $520.00 per year for international individuals, $783.00 per year for international institutions and $235.00 per year for Canadian and foreign students/residents. To receive student/resident rate, orders must be accompanied by name or affiliated institution, date of term, and the *signature* of program/residency coordinator on institution letterhead. Orders will be billed at individual rate until proof of status is received. Foreign air speed delivery is included in all *Clinics* subscription prices. All prices are subject to change without notice. **POSTMASTER:** Send address changes to *Oral and Maxillofacial Surgery Clinics of North America,* Elsevier Periodicals **Customer Service, 11830 Westline Industrial Drive, St. Louis, MO 63146. Tel: 1-800-654-2452 (U.S. and Canada); 314-447-8871 (outside U.S. and Canada). Fax: 314-447-8029. E-mail: journals customerservice-usa@elsevier.com (for print support); journalsonlinesupport-usa@elsevier.com (for online support).**

Reprints. For copies of 100 or more, of articles in this publication, please contact the Commercial Reprints Department, Elsevier Inc., 360 Park Avenue South, New York, NY 10010-1710. Tel.: 212-633-3874; Fax: 212-633-3820; Email: reprints@elsevier.com.

Oral and Maxillofacial Surgery Clinics of North America is covered in *MEDLINE/PubMed* (*Index Medicus*), *Science Citation Index Expanded (SciSearch®)*, *Journal Citation Reports/Science Edition*, and *Current Contents®/Clinical Medicine*.

Contributors

CONSULTING EDITOR

RICHARD H. HAUG, DDS
Professor and Chief, Oral Maxillofacial Surgery,
Carolinas Medical Center, Charlotte, North
Carolina

EDITOR

ALAN S. HERFORD, DDS, MD
Professor; Chair, Oral & Maxillofacial Surgery,
Loma Linda University, Loma Linda, California

AUTHORS

TARA L. AGHALOO, DDS, MD, PHD
Professor, Section of Oral and Maxillofacial
Surgery, Division of Diagnostic and Surgical
Sciences, Assistant Dean for Clinical
Research, UCLA School of Dentistry, Los
Angeles, California

SAM SEOHO BAE, DDS, MD
Senior Resident, Department of Oral and
Maxillofacial Surgery, University of Michigan
Health System, Towsley Center, Ann Arbor,
Michigan

OKSANA BUDINSKAYA, DDS
Clinical Associate Professor, Diagnostic
Sciences, Baylor College of Dentistry, Dallas,
Texas

BERNARD J. COSTELLO, DMD, MD, FACS
Professor; Associate Dean for Faculty Affairs;
Chief, Cranofacial Cleft Surgery, Department of
Oral and Maxillofacial Surgery, University of
Pittsburgh School of Dental Medicine,
Pittsburgh, Pennsylvania

**STEPHEN ELLIOTT FEINBERG, DDS, MS,
PhD**
Professor of Surgery and Dentistry; Associate
Chair of Research, Oral and Maxillofacial
Surgery, Department of Oral and Maxillofacial
Surgery, University of Michigan Health System,
Towsley Center, Ann Arbor, Michigan

DANNY HADAYA, BS
Division of Diagnostic and Surgical Sciences,
UCLA School of Dentistry, Los Angeles,
California

ALAN S. HERFORD, DDS, MD
Professor; Chair, Oral & Maxillofacial Surgery,
Loma Linda University, Loma Linda, California

F. KURTIS KASPER, PhD
Assistant Professor, Department of
Orthodontics, The University of Texas School
of Dentistry, Houston, Texas

BEOMJUNE KIM, DMD, MD, FACS
Assistant Professor, Department of Oral and
Maxillofacial Surgery, Louisiana State
University Health Sciences Center, New
Orleans, Louisiana

RODERICK YOUNGDO KIM, DDS, MD
Chief Resident, Department of Oral and
Maxillofacial Surgery, University of Michigan
Health System, Towsley Center, Ann Arbor,
Michigan

ANH D. LE, DDS, PhD
Chair and Norman-Vine Professor,
Department of Oral and Maxillofacial
Surgery/Pharmacology, University of
Pennsylvania, School of Dental Medicine,
Philadelphia, Pennsylvania

JAMES MELVILLE, DDS
Assistant Professor, Department of Oral and
Maxillofacial Surgery, The University of Texas
School of Dentistry, Houston, Texas

MEAGAN MILLER, DDS
Philip J. Boyne and Peter Geistlich Research
Intern, Oral & Maxillofacial Surgery, Loma
Linda University, Loma Linda, California

NEEL PATEL, DMD, MD
Resident, Department of Oral and Maxillofacial
Surgery, Louisiana State University Health
Sciences Center, New Orleans, Louisiana

GAURAV SHAH, DMD, MD, MPH
Resident, Department of Oral and Maxillofacial
Surgery, University of Pittsburgh School of
Dental Medicine, Pittsburgh, Pennsylvania

PASHA SHAKOORI, DDS, MA
Department of Oral and Maxillofacial Surgery/
Pharmacology, University of Pennsylvania,
School of Dental Medicine, Philadelphia,
Pennsylvania

JONATHAN SHUM, DDS, MD
Assistant Professor, Department of Oral and
Maxillofacial Surgery, The University of Texas
School of Dentistry, Houston, Texas

FABRIZIO SIGNORINO, DDS
Resident, Oral Surgery, Department of Dental
Implants, University of Milan, Milan, Italy

DANIEL SPAGNOLI, DDS, MS, PhD
Private Practice, Brunswick Oral and
Maxillofacial Surgery, Southport, North
Carolina

JAYINI S. THAKKER, DDS, MD
Assistant Professor and Residency Program
Director, Department of Oral and Maxillofacial
Surgery, Loma Linda University School of
Dentistry, Loma Linda, California

R. GILBERT TRIPLETT, DDS, PhD
Regents Professor, Department of Oral and
Maxillofacial Surgery, Texas A&M – College of
Dentistry, Chief of Division Dentistry,
Department of Surgery, Baylor University
Medical Center, Dallas, Texas

MARK WONG, DDS
Professor; Chair; Program Director;
Department of Oral and Maxillofacial Surgery,
The University of Texas School of Dentistry,
Houston, Texas

SIMON YOUNG, DDS, MD, PhD
Assistant Professor, Department of Oral and
Maxillofacial Surgery, The University of Texas
School of Dentistry, Houston, Texas

WALEED ZAID, DDS, FRCD(c), MSc
Assistant Professor, Department of Oral and
Maxillofacial Surgery, Louisiana State
University Health Sciences Center, New
Orleans, Louisiana

KIROLLOS E. ZAKHARY, DDS, MD
Resident, Oral and Maxillofacial Surgery, Loma
Linda University, Loma Linda, California

QUANZHOU ZHANG, PhD
Department of Oral and Maxillofacial Surgery/
Pharmacology, University of Pennsylvania,
School of Dental Medicine, Philadelphia,
Pennsylvania

CONTENTS

In a quest to provide best-quality treatment, results, and long-term prognosis, physicians must be well versed in emerging sciences and discoveries to more favorably provide suitable options to patients. Bioengineering and regeneration have rapidly developed, and with them, the options afforded to surgeons are ever-expanding. Grafting techniques can be modified according to evolving knowledge. The basic principles of bioengineering are discussed in this article to provide a solid foundation for favorable treatment and a comprehensive understanding of the reasons why each particular treatment available can be the most adequate for each particular case.

Soft tissue replacement and repair is crucial to the ever-developing field of reconstructive surgery as trauma, pathology, and congenital deficits cannot be adequately restored if soft tissue regeneration is deficient. Predominant approaches were sometimes limited to harvesting autografts, but through regenerative medicine and tissue engineering, the hope of fabricating custom constructs is now a feasible and fast-approaching reality. The breadth of this field includes tissues ranging from skin, mucosa, muscle, and fat and hopes to not only provide construct to replace a tissue but also to replace its function.

The field of tissue engineering and regenerative medicine has been rapidly expanded through multidisciplinary integration of research and clinical practice in response to unmet clinical needs for reconstruction of dental, oral, and craniofacial structures. The significance of the various types of stem cells, specifically mesenchymal stem cells derived from the orofacial tissues, ranging from dental pulp stem cells to periodontal ligament stem cells to mucosa/gingiva has been thoroughly investigated and their applications in tissue regeneration are outlined in this article.

This article provides an overview of basic tissue engineering principles as they are applied to vertical ridge defects and reconstructive techniques for these types of deficiencies. Presented are multiple clinical cases ranging from office-based dentoalveolar procedures to the more complex reconstruction of postresection mandibular defects. Several different types of regenerative tissue constructs are presented; either used alone or in combination with traditional reconstructive techniques and procedures, such as maxillary sinus augmentation, Le Fort I osteotomy, and microvascular free tissue transfer. The goal is to also familiarize the reconstructive surgeon to potential future strategies in vertical alveolar ridge augmentation.

 Video content accompanies this article at http://www.oralmaxsurgery.theclinics.com.

Emerging technologies and research into the science of biomaterials have developed exponentially and provide facial reconstructive surgeons with a plethora of options for a multitude of varying presentations. This article presents a comprehensive discussion in the ever-evolving field of material science and emerging biomaterials. A complete understanding of the current status of such materials is necessary for the appropriate incorporation and applicability to adequate clinical situations. The rapid progress seen in biomaterials is evidenced through the forward direction of bioengineered tissues, the incorporation of growth factors in varying scenarios, and the unique characteristics of 3-D printing of patient specific scaffolds.

The complex shapes of skeletal components of the craniofacial region combined with the prominence of the face and paucity of overlying soft tissue create significant challenges for the reconstructive surgeon. The in vivo bioreactor strategy is a promising alternative to microvascular surgical techniques that combines tissue engineering principles with microvascular reconstructive techniques to create patient-specific, prevascularized bone flaps for reconstruction of complex maxillofacial defects. This article discusses the use of traditional vascularized bone flaps; preclinical studies using the in vivo bioreactor approach; case reports that have attempted this novel technique; and future challenges and considerations in the development of patient-specific, prevascularized bone flaps for maxillofacial reconstruction.

The development and increase in knowledge of the benefits and applications of growth factors in craniofacial reconstruction adds a novel tool in the reconstructive surgeon's armamentarium. The use of growth factors varies according to presentation. Growth factors help to promote healing, angiogenesis, and formation of bone of improved quality and quantity. Growth factors used with stem cells and scaffolds provide a solution or alternative to discomfort created by donor autograft sites. The application and results of these growth factors are displayed in various examples of maxillofacial defects in this article, including reconstruction of a premaxillary cleft and of maxillary augmentation.

There is a recognized need to reconstruct and restore complex craniomaxillofacial soft tissues. The objective of this article is to focus on the role that tissue engineering/regenerative medicine can play in addressing various barriers (vascularity, tissue bulk, volitional control, and esthetics) and impediments (timing, regional applicability/dissemination, and regulation by the US Food and Drug Administration) to optimal tissue reconstruction of complex soft tissue structures. We will use the lips as an example to illustrate our points.

New Frontiers in Biomaterials 105

R. Gilbert Triplett and Oksana Budinskaya

Scientific and technological advances have combined to lead the way into a new era of the ever-developing science of biomaterials and tissue regeneration. This field has rapidly grown and new frontiers have quickly been established. Despite obtaining satisfactory results with current methods, improved techniques that lead to diminished patient discomfort, more favorable long-term prognosis, and decreased health care costs continue to be the goals of researchers, patients, and surgeons. Biomaterials have undergone a rapid evolution from materials that simply replaced tissues to factors that stimulate a biological response in the body.

Index 117

ORAL AND MAXILLOFACIAL SURGERY CLINICS OF NORTH AMERICA

Preface
Regeneration and Beyond

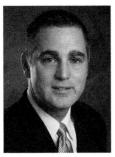

Alan S. Herford, DDS, MD, FACS
Editor

Reconstructive craniomaxillofacial surgery has evolved exponentially, and today's patients can benefit from treatment that years ago was thought impossible. The collaboration of researchers, patients, and surgeons has enabled the fast development in the field of biomaterials and the improvement and evolution of techniques in tissue regeneration. The present possibilities of treatment and the future outlook provide numerous solutions for existing treatment challenges and innumerable opportunities for the continued development in this field.

With the advancement of technology, the integration of research, and the observations of clinical trials, limitations in previous therapies have been overcome and new boundaries are continuously being set. Initially, the use of biomaterials in the therapy of reconstruction was limited to just that—materials that would simply replace a missing tissue. Today, the use and combination of new biomaterials allow the replacement construct to actually stimulate a biological response from the host. This in turn results in more favorable integration and better long-term prognosis.

This issue begins with an overview of the ever-evolving new frontiers of biomaterials, detailing existing therapies, current research, and potential developments in the field of both novel biomaterials and tissue regeneration. The basic principles are discussed in the initial articles.

Advances in stem cell research, specifically orofacial stem cells, have had huge implications in the overall development and refinement of previous therapies. Simultaneous advances in the research of growth factors, scaffold systems, and 3D printing have allowed for all of these components to be combined, evaluated, and improved, leading to the fabrication of continuously refined constructs that have become a foundational part of reconstructive surgery. The ultimate goal of craniomaxillofacial reconstruction is not only to restore missing tissues but also to do so in a manner that most closely mimics the natural state in both form and function.

The integration of the innovative biomaterials and tissue regeneration techniques is displayed in this issue through various cases ranging from soft tissue regeneration to tissue engineered prevascularized bone flaps.

Through the collaboration of the leaders in their respective fields, this issue encompasses the many aspects of emerging biomaterials and the techniques in tissue regeneration. It is the goal of this collaboration to provide invaluable information through both research and clinical examples that will be beneficial to oral and maxillofacial surgeons that will ultimately lead the way in the continued path to the refinement of biomaterials and tissue regeneration.

Alan S. Herford, DDS, MD, FACS
Department of Oral and Maxillofacial Surgery
Loma Linda University School of Dentistry
11092 Anderson Street
Loma Linda, CA 92350, USA

E-mail address:
aherford@llu.edu

Oral Maxillofacial Surg Clin N Am 29 (2017) ix
http://dx.doi.org/10.1016/j.coms.2016.10.001
1042-3699/17/© 2016 Published by Elsevier Inc.

oralmaxsurgery.theclinics.com

Basic Principles of Bioengineering and Regeneration

Tara L. Aghaloo, DDS, MD, PhD[a],*, Danny Hadaya, BS[b]

KEYWORDS

- Autogenous grafts • Allografts • Osteoinductive • Osteoconductive • Scaffolds • Stem cells
- Growth factors • Angiogenesis

KEY POINTS

- Research into fabricating allografts may potentially reduce the need for autografts, thus reducing donor site morbidity.
- Different systems of delivery of stem cells have been explored with varying results.
- The use of growth factors along with stem cells and scaffolding systems has been shown to aid in grafting procedures.

INTRODUCTION

Although wound healing in the oral cavity occurs with minimal scarring, and oral tissue repair can take place in conditions of dental disease and infection, complex hard and soft tissue defects pose major challenges to clinicians and researchers.[1] Current methods range from simple autogenous or alloplast bone grafting to the use of growth factors with stem cells supported by biodegradable scaffolds to create elaborate 3-D constructs for tissue regeneration.[2–6] Although autogenous bone is the gold standard grafting material due to its osteogenic, osteoinductive, and osteoconductive properties, it has significant drawbacks, including a second surgical site with associated morbidity and resorption over time.[7–10] Bone graft substitutes, such as allografts, xenografts, and alloplasts, are a constant source of investigation with the goal of retaining the favorable characteristics of autogenous grafts without donor site morbidity.[11–13] Unfortunately, bone substitutes lack significant osteoinductive properties and autogenous bone grafts often create unacceptable donor site morbidity to reconstruct large or challenging craniomaxillofacial defects. Therefore, the search for methods to repair and regenerate missing or damaged craniofacial structures rather than grafting or reconstructing them is the ultimate goal of current and future research.

It is widely known that the human body has the capacity to regenerate certain tissues, such as the liver, which can regain function after significant loss.[14] Hepatocytes and liver parenchyma replicate and repopulate the missing area, restoring it to full function.[15] Unfortunately, this process of regeneration does not occur in the oral cavity or elsewhere in the body. If any oral soft or hard tissue is lost, it does not return to its original form. Instead, repair occurs, where damaged tissue is replaced by a fibrous network, without restoration in form or function.[16] Therefore, regeneration must take place by grafting hard and/or soft tissue.

Disclosure Statement: The authors have nothing to disclose.
[a] Section of Oral and Maxillofacial Surgery, Division of Diagnostic and Surgical Sciences, School of Dentistry, University of California, Los Angeles, 10833 Le Conte Avenue, CHS 53-076, Los Angeles, CA 90095, USA;
[b] Division of Diagnostic and Surgical Sciences, School of Dentistry, University of California, Los Angeles, 10833 Le Conte Avenue, CHS 53-076, Los Angeles, CA 90095, USA
* Correspondence author.
E-mail address: taghaloo@dentistry.ucla.edu

Currently, more than 1 million bone grafts are performed each year in the United States,[11] which puts a large economic burden on the health care system. Decreasing invasiveness of the procedures and eliminating the need for harvesting donor tissue, while continuing to improve outcomes are major goals for tissue engineering. As researchers become more successful with stem cell isolation and differentiation, developing improved scaffolds that are able to stimulate multiple tissue types while supporting vascularity and producing growth factors that can attain Food and Drug Administration (FDA) approval, the field of tissue engineering will continue to advance and tackle new challenges in tissue repair and regeneration.

BIOLOGICAL MECHANISMS OF WOUND REGENERATION AND REPAIR

The process of regeneration and repair begins with the formation of a wound. This leads to an inflammatory cascade that activates hemostasis. Platelets help to form an initial barrier from the outside environment and secrete growth factors from their α-granules.[17] Fibrinogen, a soluble protein, is converted into fibrin, an insoluble protein that creates a solid clot and provides a scaffold for further inflammatory cells.[18] Various cells in the environment, after being stimulated by injury, secrete chemotactic factors, such as platelet-derived growth factor (PDGF), epidermal growth factor, histamine, and von Willebrand factor.[19] The combination of these signals attracts macrophages and other leukocytes to the area, which destroy bacteria and decontaminate the area, ending the inflammatory portion of the process.[16]

The proliferation phase is marked by angiogenesis and the formation of fibrous tissue during this process; the tissue volume is re-established by fibrous repair.[20] Growth factors released from early cells in the healing wound, such as PDGF, transforming growth factor β-1 (TGF-β1), vascular endothelial growth factor (VEGF), insulin-like growth factor, basic fibroblast growth factor, and epidermal growth factor from macrophages and platelets, are responsible for beginning angiogenesis and vasculogenesis.[21,22] New blood vessels form in the granulation tissue and begin the reconstruction of the area.

After this proliferative phase, the wounded tissue undergoes remodeling and maturation. Myofibroblasts, a combination of smooth muscle cells and fibroblasts, contract to close the wound. Collagen fibers become more organized and the epithelium over the area is regenerated.[2,23] Current methods used to regenerate tissue target various portions of this pathway to achieve a desirable result, yet unfortunately the tensile strength of the healed tissue is not equal to the uninjured tissue.[24,25]

BASIC PRINCIPLES OF BONE HEALING

Missing hard tissue in the craniofacial region or oral cavity can be augmented through various procedures, each of which has benefits and pitfalls. Regardless of the material or method used, all these techniques have a few basic principles that must be followed. Many of these techniques are based on cell exclusion and cellular proliferation.[26] Cell exclusion involves the use of a resorbable or nonresorbable membrane to limit the ingrowth of epithelial cells. Cellular proliferation is the differentiation and growth of cells in response to a certain stimulus. The success of regeneration is greatly dependent on the vascular supply available in the area. Because of this, biomaterials are frequently combined with angiogenesis stimulators.[27]

Bone augmentation is an attempt to preserve or regain bone in preparation for a prosthesis, whether an implant or denture. Various techniques are currently reported in the literature, but they all follow the same principles.[28] After extraction, it is a widely known fact that alveolar bone undergoes marked atrophy. Approximately 3.8 mm of bone is lost horizontally, whereas 1.2 mm is lost vertically.[29] To prevent this resorption, extraction socket augmentation or preservation is often performed. This procedure is generally simple and only requires particulate grafting material to serve as a scaffold to prevent soft tissue ingrowth and significantly reduces the horizontal and vertical resorption compared with tooth extraction alone.[30] Biomaterials include autografts, allografts, xenografts, and synthetic alloplasts.[31] The most commonly used materials are bovine-derived xenografts, which have proved clinically effective.[32]

Bone augmentation relies on 3 mechanisms: osteogenesis, osteoinduction, and osteoconduction. Osteogenesis involves the transplantation of osteocompetent cells to the recipient site. Only autogenous bone has osteogenic properties, especially trabecular bone with more bone marrow and increased cellularity. This is why the iliac crest is a preferred site for large craniofacial defects. Both anterior and posterior approaches provide cortical and cancellous bone and have been successful for continuity defects, alveolar clefts, and severe alveolar atrophy.[3,4,13] Osteoinduction involves chemotaxis of undifferentiated mesenchymal stem cells to the recipient site and stimulates them to become osteoblasts and form bone. Autogenous bone and specific bone morphogenic proteins (BMPs) possess osteoinductive properties.

Certain demineralized allografts may have weak osteoinductive properties, but these are entirely dependent on donor variability.[33] Osteoconduction is the graft's ability to provide a scaffold, or surface, for the formation of new bone, which can be provided by most commercially available bone substitutes, including xenografts, allografts, and alloplasts. Together these mechanisms provide the formation of a stable, integrated, and vital bone structure.[2,4,34–37]

GROWTH FACTORS

The use of growth factors for tissue regeneration depends on the ability of these exogenous signals to stimulate a patient's own cells and immune system. Growth factors are secreted by multiple cell types in both temporal and spatial patterns for normal wound healing. Although wound healing is a complex process and requires multiple cells, growth factors, vascularity, and fibrin networks, clinicians and researchers are using specific growth factors to aid in bone and soft tissue repair and regeneration.[38] Because recapitulating natural wound healing is a goal of reconstructive and regenerative medicine, growth factors will definitely play a major role in current and future clinical oral and maxillofacial surgery. Although years and perhaps even decades of work have yet to be done, there has been significant progress in the field that has left commercially available recombinant growth factors and platelet concentrates to aid in the wound-healing process. The most potent osteoinductive growth factor, BMP-2, is already FDA approved on an absorbable collagen sponge for use in spinal fusion surgery and for nonunion of tibial fractures. Since 2007, BMP-2 is also approved for maxillary sinus augmentation and localized alveolar ridge defects associated with extraction sites.[39–43] BMP-2 is chemotactic for undifferentiated mesenchymal stem cells, and up-regulates VEGF to enhance angiogenesis.[44] PDGF is the other molecule that is approved for use in dentistry, where the recombinant factor is combined with a β-tricalcium phosphate carrier for use in intrabony periodontal defects and for gingival recession.[45,46] PDGF, however, is most effective in enhancing vascularity, where it has been extremely successful in treating diabetic foot ulcers.[47,48]

Platelet concentrates, such as platelet-rich plasma and platelet-rich fibrin, are extremely popular in many surgical fields to decrease bleeding and swelling as well as aid in wound healing. Because multiple growth factors in the platelet α-granules promote vascularity, angiogenesis, enhance fibroblast proliferation, collagen synthesis, and extracellular matrix production, endothelial cell proliferation, the impetus to use platelet concentrates in bone and soft tissue grafting for enhanced tissue regeneration is well understood.[37,49,50] Few definitive studies can document significant effects on bone and soft tissue regeneration using platelet concentrates, however, thus questioning their routine use. Wound-healing adjuncts are tremendously desirable, which makes clinicians, researchers, and even patients the driving forces behind their use. The question remains if they significantly enhance wound healing and regeneration, and if they should be used in all patients as opposed to patients with compromised healing.

DISTRACTION OSTEOGENESIS

Distraction osteogenesis (DO) is a technique that creates a bone fracture and then applies a mechanical stress to stimulate bone formation.[51] In oral and maxillofacial surgery, the technique is often used to advance a retrognathic mandible or maxilla, especially in cleft palate patients or patients with significant craniofacial anomalies.[52] DO functions differently from a bone graft because it uses the principles of tension from 2 osteotomized vascular bone surfaces and the importance of neovascularization.[4,53] When the bone segments separate gradually after a latency period allows for blood clot formation, new bone forms mainly through intramembranous ossification after vessels grow on either side of the fibrous callous adjacent to osteoid tissue.[54–56] The role of the vasculature is so important that rats treated with angiogenic inhibitors had nonunion of the distracted bone segments.[57] Growth factors also play a major role in distraction; where BMP-2 and BMP-4 are expressed during the early latency stage, TGF-β is expressed until the consolidation stage, and VEGF is responsible for neovascularization.[4,58] Although DO has similar bone healing characteristics of a fracture model, DO has some complications and limitations that may prevent its widespread and routine use. Both craniofacial and alveolar distraction require patient and/or parent compliance, pose challenges controlling the vector of movement, may fail to form a uniform bone regenerate, may develop infection or inflammation from the distraction pin, and are susceptible to relapse.

SOFT TISSUE REGENERATION

Although major progress has been made in hard tissue engineering where growth factors, scaffolds, and cells are used in patients with small and large craniofacial defects, soft tissue engineering lags significantly behind.[59] Over the past decades, free gingival and connective tissue grafts have been used in clinical dentistry to treat gingival recession, increase keratinized tissue, and augment missing tissue. Soft tissue is harvested, usually from the palate, and has become highly predictable in providing patients with an esthetic solution to common mucogingival problems.[60–62] Just like for all other autogenous tissue transfers with unwanted donor site morbidity, however, a search for alternative solutions is present.

Collagen matrices are available alternatives that can be used to augment oral soft tissue deficiencies around teeth and dental implants.[63–65] These collagen matrices are treated like gingival or subepithelial connective tissue but are a nonautogenous tissue substitute. Although they have some preliminarily favorable results, the success is limited to small and simple defects. To regenerate larger and more complex volumes of soft tissue, tissue engineering principles must be followed.[59] Preliminary clinical reports as well as multiple animal studies demonstrate the development of an ex vivo–produced oral mucosal equivalent that consists of a patient's own keratinocytes cultured on a commercially available acellular freeze-dried dermis stimulated by signaling molecules in the culture media.[59,66–69] These data are particularly exciting because soft tissue defects are extremely challenging to treat, especially because they are exposed to the oral cavity with risk of contamination and infection.

STEM CELLS

Stem cell therapy has had a major impact on medicine and surgery over the past decade. In the dental field, specifically oral and maxillofacial surgery, bone marrow mesenchymal cells have been used for many years as bone marrow aspirate.[70–72] In addition, the ability to isolate and culture stem cells from dental origin, including dental pulp stem cells, stem cells from apical papilla, maxillary and mandibular bone marrow, and stem cells from exfoliated deciduous teeth that can differentiate into multiple cell types, makes the future of regenerating entire craniofacial structures seem attainable.[73–75] Stem cells are immature, undifferentiated cells that, when given the proper signals, can differentiate into any type of cell.[76] Studies in animal models already demonstrate that pulpal stem cells have the ability to regenerate alveolar bone defects.[77] Although whole-tooth regeneration is still an abstract concept, bioengineered teeth have successfully

been created and implanted into pigs.[78] This new concept of stem cell differentiation and functioning regenerated tissue shows that using bioengineering to recreate missing hard and soft tissue is not far off.

SUMMARY

Bioengineering has opened the door for countless abstract ideas to rehabilitate the oral cavity and entire craniofacial structure. Clinically, there are numerous successful and predictable procedures that are used to augment and regenerate missing hard and soft tissue. Improving these current techniques, however, specifically by decreasing or omitting the need for autogenous grafts, is the ultimate goal of clinicians and researchers. This cannot be attained unless new technologies are equivalent or superior to the gold standard of autogenous tissue. The attempt to recapitulate the complex wound-healing process of bringing the appropriate cells to the wound site that can secrete or stimulate the required growth factors with spatial and temporal precision, all on a biodegradable matrix, is an extremely challenging order. Nevertheless, the rewards of this objective cannot be overstated, and these continue to stimulate scientists all over the world to strive for success. This articles describe the past, present, and future of biomaterials and techniques in tissue regeneration and how oral and maxillofacial surgeons play a major role in helping the field progress.

REFERENCES

1. Teven CM, Fisher S, Ameer GA, et al. Biomimetic approaches to complex craniofacial defects. Ann Maxillofac Surg 2015;5(1):4–13.
2. Aghaloo TL, Felsenfeld AL. Principles of repair and grafting of bone and cartilage. In: Bagheri S, Bell R, Khan H, editors. Current therapy in oral and maxillofacial surgery. St Louis (MO): Elsevier; 2012.
3. Costello BJ, Kumta P, Sfeir CS. Regenerative technologies for craniomaxillofacial surgery. J Oral Maxillofac Surg 2015;73(12 Suppl):S116–25.
4. Fishero BA, Kohli N, Das A, et al. Current concepts of bone tissue engineering for craniofacial bone defect repair. Craniomaxillofac Trauma Reconstr 2015;8(1):23–30.
5. Tevlin R, McArdle A, Atashroo D, et al. Biomaterials for craniofacial bone engineering. J Dent Res 2014;93(12):1187–95.
6. Larsson L, Decker AM, Nibali L, et al. Regenerative medicine for periodontal and peri-implant diseases. J Dent Res 2015;95:255–66.
7. Janicki P, Schmidmaier G. What should be the characteristics of the ideal bone graft substitute?

Combining scaffolds with growth factors and/or stem cells. Injury 2011;42(Suppl 2):S77–81.

8. Keating JF, McQueen MM. Substitutes for autologous bone graft in orthopaedic trauma. J Bone Joint Surg Br 2001;83(1):3–8.

9. Finkemeier CG. Bone-grafting and bone-graft substitutes. J Bone Joint Surg Am 2002;84-A(3):454–64.

10. Chiapasco M, Zaniboni M. Failures in jaw reconstructive surgery with autogenous onlay bone grafts for pre-implant purposes: incidence, prevention and management of complications. Oral Maxillofac Surg Clin North Am 2011;23(1):1–15, v.

11. Gruskin E, Doll BA, Futrell FW, et al. Demineralized bone matrix in bone repair: history and use. Adv Drug Deliv Rev 2012;64(12):1063–77.

12. Acocella A, Bertolai R, Ellis E 3rd, et al. Maxillary alveolar ridge reconstruction with monocortical fresh-frozen bone blocks: a clinical, histological and histomorphometric study. J Craniomaxillofac Surg 2012;40(6):525–33.

13. Aghaloo TL, Moy PK. Which hard tissue augmentation techniques are the most successful in furnishing bony support for implant placement? Int J Oral Maxillofac Implants 2007;22(Suppl):49–70.

14. Stoltz JF, de Isla N, Li YP, et al. Stem cells and regenerative medicine: myth or reality of the 21th century. Stem Cells Int 2015;2015:734731.

15. Fausto N, Campbell JS, Riehle KJ. Liver regeneration. Hepatology 2006;43(2 Suppl 1):S45–53.

16. Clark R. Wound repair: overview and general considerations. The molecular biology of wound repair. New York: Plenum Press; 1996.

17. Werner S, Grose R. Regulation of wound healing by growth factors and cytokines. Physiol Rev 2003; 83(3):835–70.

18. Lord ST. Fibrinogen and fibrin: scaffold proteins in hemostasis. Curr Opin Hematol 2007;14(3): 236–41.

19. Heldin CH, Westermark B. Mechanism of action and in vivo role of platelet-derived growth factor. Physiol Rev 1999;79(4):1283–316.

20. Mahdavian Delavary B, van der Veer WM, van Egmond M, et al. Macrophages in skin injury and repair. Immunobiology 2011;216(7):753–62.

21. Schliephake H. Clinical efficacy of growth factors to enhance tissue repair in oral and maxillofacial reconstruction: a systematic review. Clin Implant Dent Relat Res 2015;17(2):247–73.

22. Harrison P, Cramer EM. Platelet alpha-granules. Blood Rev 1993;7(1):52–62.

23. Wynn T. Common and unique mechanisms regulate fibrosis in various fibroproliferative diseases. J Clin Invest 2007;117(3):524–9.

24. Schilling JA. Wound healing. Surg Clin North Am 1976;56(4):859–74.

25. Xue M, Jackson CJ. Extracellular matrix reorganization during wound healing and its impact on abnormal scarring. Adv Wound Care (New Rochelle) 2015;4(3):119–36.

26. Gentile P, Chiono V, Tonda-Turo C, et al. Polymeric membranes for guided bone regeneration. Biotechnol J 2011;6(10):1187–97.

27. Oh SH, Kim TH, Chun SY, et al. Enhanced guided bone regeneration by asymmetrically porous PCL/ pluronic F127 membrane and ultrasound stimulation. J Biomater Sci Polym Ed 2012;23(13):1673–86.

28. Guiol J, Campard G, Longis J, et al. Anterior mandibular bone augmentation techniques. Literature review. Rev Stomatol Chir Maxillofac Chir Orale 2015;116(6):353–9 [in French].

29. Tan WL, Wong TL, Wong MC, et al. A systematic review of post-extractional alveolar hard and soft tissue dimensional changes in humans. Clin Oral Implants Res 2012;23(Suppl 5):1–21.

30. Avila-Ortiz G, Elangovan S, Kramer KW, et al. Effect of alveolar ridge preservation after tooth extraction: a systematic review and meta-analysis. J Dent Res 2014;93(10):950–8.

31. Eppley BL, Pietrzak WS, Blanton MW. Allograft and alloplastic bone substitutes: a review of science and technology for the craniomaxillofacial surgeon. J Craniofac Surg 2005;16(6):981–9.

32. Richardson CR, Mellonig JT, Brunsvold MA, et al. Clinical evaluation of bio-oss: a bovine-derived xenograft for the treatment of periodontal osseous defects in humans. J Clin Periodontol 1999;26(7): 421–8.

33. Boyan BD, Ranly DM, Schwartz Z. Use of growth factors to modify osteoinductivity of demineralized bone allografts: lessons for tissue engineering of bone. Dent Clin North Am 2006;50(2):217–28, viii.

34. Siddiqui NA, Owen JM. Clinical advances in bone regeneration. Curr Stem Cell Res Ther 2013;8(3): 192–200.

35. Roberts TT, Rosenbaum AJ. Bone grafts, bone substitutes and orthobiologics: the bridge between basic science and clinical advancements in fracture healing. Organogenesis 2012;8(4):114–24.

36. Einhorn TA. The cell and molecular biology of fracture healing. Clin Orthop Relat Res 1998; 355(Suppl):S7–21.

37. Ulma R, Aghaloo TL, Freymiller E. Wound healing. In: Fonseca R, HD B, Powers M, et al, editors. Oral and maxillofacial trauma. St. Louis (MO): Elsevier; 2013. p. 9.

38. Aghaloo TL, Pi-Anfruns J, Simel O, et al. Growth factors in implant dentistry. In: Moy P, Beumer J, Shah K, editors. Fundamentals of implant dentistry. Chicago: Quintessence; 2016.

39. Boyne PJ, Lilly LC, Marx RE, et al. De novo bone induction by recombinant human bone morphogenetic protein-2 (rhBMP-2) in maxillary sinus floor augmentation. J Oral Maxillofac Surg 2005;63(12): 1693–707.

40. Triplett RG, Nevins M, Marx RE, et al. Pivotal, randomized, parallel evaluation of recombinant human bone morphogenetic protein-2/absorbable collagen sponge and autogenous bone graft for maxillary sinus floor augmentation. J Oral Maxillofac Surg 2009;67(9):1947–60.

41. Fiorellini JP, Howell TH, Cochran D, et al. Randomized study evaluating recombinant human bone morphogenetic protein-2 for extraction socket augmentation. J Periodontol 2005;76(4):605–13.

42. Wozney JM. Overview of bone morphogenetic proteins. Spine (Phila Pa 1976) 2002;27(16 Suppl 1): S2–8.

43. Yamaguchi A, Komori T, Suda T. Regulation of osteoblast differentiation mediated by bone morphogenetic proteins, hedgehogs, and Cbfa1. Endocr Rev 2000;21(4):393–411.

44. Spagnoli DB, Marx RE. Dental implants and the use of rhBMP-2. Oral Maxillofac Surg Clin North Am 2011;23(2):347–61, vii.

45. Nevins M, Giannobile WV, McGuire MK, et al. Platelet-derived growth factor stimulates bone fill and rate of attachment level gain: results of a large multicenter randomized controlled trial. J Periodontol 2005;76(12):2205–15.

46. Howell TH, Fiorellini JP, Paquette DW, et al. A phase I/II clinical trial to evaluate a combination of recombinant human platelet-derived growth factor-BB and recombinant human insulin-like growth factor-I in patients with periodontal disease. J Periodontol 1997;68(12):1186–93.

47. Steed DL. Clinical evaluation of recombinant human platelet-derived growth factor for the treatment of lower extremity ulcers. Plast Reconstr Surg 2006; 117(7 Suppl):143S–9S [discussion: 150S–1S].

48. Wieman TJ, Smiell JM, Su Y. Efficacy and safety of a topical gel formulation of recombinant human platelet-derived growth factor-BB (becaplermin) in patients with chronic neuropathic diabetic ulcers. A phase III randomized placebo-controlled double-blind study. Diabetes Care 1998;21(5):822–7.

49. Barrientos S, Stojadinovic O, Golinko MS, et al. Growth factors and cytokines in wound healing. Wound Repair Regen 2008;16(5):585–601.

50. Marx RE. Platelet-rich plasma: a source of multiple autologous growth factors for bone grafts. In: Lynch SE, Genco RJ, Marx RE, editors. Tissue Engineering: applications in maxillofacial surgery and periodontics. Chicago: Quintessence; 1999. p. 71.

51. Dhaliwal K, Kunchur R, Farhadieh R. Review of the cellular and biological principles of distraction osteogenesis: an in vivo bioreactor tissue engineering model. J Plast Reconstr Aesthet Surg 2016;69: e19–26.

52. Chin M. The role of distraction osteogenesis in oral and maxillofacial surgery. J Oral Maxillofac Surg 1998;56(6):805–6.

53. Ai-Aql ZS, Alagl AS, Graves DT, et al. Molecular mechanisms controlling bone formation during fracture healing and distraction osteogenesis. J Dent Res 2008;87(2):107–18.

54. Aronson J, Good B, Stewart C, et al. Preliminary studies of mineralization during distraction osteogenesis. Clin Orthop Relat Res 1990;(250):43–9.

55. Delloye C, Delefortrie G, Coutelier L, et al. Bone regenerate formation in cortical bone during distraction lengthening. An experimental study. Clin Orthop Relat Res 1990;(250):34–42.

56. Percival CJ, Richtsmeier JT. Angiogenesis and intramembranous osteogenesis. Dev Dyn 2013;242(8): 909–22.

57. Fang TD, Salim A, Xia W, et al. Angiogenesis is required for successful bone induction during distraction osteogenesis. J Bone Miner Res 2005; 20(7):1114–24.

58. Choi IH, Chung CY, Cho TJ, et al. Angiogenesis and mineralization during distraction osteogenesis. J Korean Med Sci 2002;17(4):435–47.

59. Kim RY, Fasi AC, Feinberg SE. Soft tissue engineering in craniomaxillofacial surgery. Ann Maxillofac Surg 2014;4(1):4–8.

60. Shah R, Thomas R, Mehta DS. Recent modifications of free gingival graft: a case series. Contemp Clin Dent 2015;6(3):425–7.

61. Bassetti RG, Stähli A, Bassetti MA, et al. Soft tissue augmentation procedures at second-stage surgery: a systematic review. Clin Oral Investig 2016;20: 1369–87.

62. Thoma DS, Buranawat B, Hämmerle CH, et al. Efficacy of soft tissue augmentation around dental implants and in partially edentulous areas: a systematic review. J Clin Periodontol 2014;41(Suppl 15): S77–91.

63. Thoma DS, Zeltner M, Hilbe M, et al. Randomized controlled clinical study evaluating effectiveness and safety of a volume-stable collagen matrix compared to autogenous connective tissue grafts for soft tissue augmentation at implant sites. J Clin Periodontol 2016;43:874–85.

64. McGuire MK, Scheyer ET. Long-term results comparing xenogeneic collagen matrix and autogenous connective tissue grafts with coronally advanced flaps for treatment of dehiscence-type recession defects. J Periodontol 2016;87(3): 221–7.

65. McGuire MK, Scheyer ET. Randomized, controlled clinical trial to evaluate a xenogeneic collagen matrix as an alternative to free gingival grafting for oral soft tissue augmentation. J Periodontol 2014; 85(10):1333–41.

66. Izumi K, Song J, Feinberg SE. Development of a tissue-engineered human oral mucosa: from the bench to the bed side. Cells Tissues Organs 2004; 176(1–3):134–52.

67. Izumi K, Feinberg SE. Skin and oral mucosal substitutes. Oral Maxillofac Surg Clin North Am 2002; 14(1):61–71.

68. Peramo A, Marcelo CL, Feinberg SE. Tissue engineering of lips and muco-cutaneous junctions: in vitro development of tissue engineered constructs of oral mucosa and skin for lip reconstruction. Tissue Eng Part C Methods 2012;18(4):273–82.

69. Izumi K, Terashi H, Marcelo CL, et al. Development and characterization of a tissue-engineered human oral mucosa equivalent produced in a serum-free culture system. J Dent Res 2000;79(3):798–805.

70. Marx RE, Harrell DB. Translational research: The CD34+ cell is crucial for large-volume bone regeneration from the milieu of bone marrow progenitor cells in craniomandibular reconstruction. Int J Oral Maxillofac Implants 2014;29(2):e201–9.

71. Soltan M, Smiler DG, Gailani F. A new "platinum" standard for bone grafting: autogenous stem cells. Implant Dent 2005;14(4):322–5.

72. Smiler DG, Soltan M, Soltan C, et al. Growth factors and gene expression of stem cells: bone marrow compared with peripheral blood. Implant Dent 2010;19(3):229–40.

73. Zhao H, Chai Y. Stem cells in teeth and craniofacial bones. J Dent Res 2015;94(11):1495–501.

74. Sakai VT, Zhang Z, Dong Z, et al. SHED differentiate into functional odontoblasts and endothelium. J Dent Res 2010;89(8):791–6.

75. Akintoye SO, Lam T, Shi S, et al. Skeletal site-specific characterization of orofacial and iliac crest human bone marrow stromal cells in same individuals. Bone 2006;38(6):758–68.

76. Girlovanu M, Susman S, Soritau O, et al. Stem cells - biological update and cell therapy progress. Clujul Med 2015;88(3):265–71.

77. Huojia M, Wu Z, Zhang X, et al. Effect of Dental Pulp Stem Cells (DPSCs) in repairing rabbit alveolar bone defect. Clin Lab 2015;61(11):1703–8.

78. Yang KC, Kitamura Y, Wu CC, et al. Tooth germ-like construct transplantation for whole-tooth regeneration: an in vivo study in the miniature pig. Artif Organs 2016;40:E39–50.

Soft Tissue Regeneration Incorporating 3-Dimensional Biomimetic Scaffolds

Gaurav Shah, DMD, MD, MPH[a],
Bernard J. Costello, DMD, MD[b],*

KEYWORDS

- Soft tissue engineering • Computer-aided design/computer-aided manufacturing
- 3-dimensional printing • Scaffolds

KEY POINTS

- Soft tissue regeneration in the craniomaxillofacial region is a burgeoning field of study. With the loss of skin, muscle, oral mucosa, or the neurovascular bundle, the predominant approach for closure has been to harvest local, regional, or distant flaps. Regenerative medicine and tissue engineering hope to provide custom constructs that become integrated fully in the local anatomy and provide ideal form and function once they are fully integrated into the host.
- Soft tissue regeneration has found momentum in reconstructing skin, oral mucosa, muscle, fat, and other soft tissue structures.
- By combining soft tissue cell lines, growth factors such as platelet-derived growth factor and transforming growth factor $\beta1$ found in sources like platelet-rich plasma, and scaffolds by virtue of 3-dimensional printing have shown promise in the field of soft tissue regeneration to develop constructs that not only obturate defects but also restore form and function.

INTRODUCTION

Soft tissue regeneration in the craniomaxillofacial region is a burgeoning field of study. Over the last 20 years, success at various centers across the world in craniomaxillofacial allotransplantation has led to more interest in developing a hybrid model of allotransplantation with tissue engineering models consisting of cell lines, biomimetic scaffolds, and biochemical signals.[1] With the loss of skin, muscle, oral mucosa, or the neurovascular bundle, the predominant approach for closure has been to harvest local, regional, or distant flaps—this technique may accomplish the closure of dead space but still lacks providing good facial function and esthetics in complex regions such as the lips or eyelids.[2] As with bone regeneration, specialists are looking for substitutes to flap reconstruction to avoid donor site morbidity in the setting of trauma, deformities, or pathologic conditions.[3] Major obstacles in soft tissue regeneration include developing and sustaining a vascular supply to the engineered construct[2] as well as immunosuppression and tissue interactions.[1] Regenerative medicine and tissue

Disclosure Statement: The authors have nothing to disclose.
[a] Department of Oral and Maxillofacial Surgery, University of Pittsburgh School of Dental Medicine, 214 Eye and Ear Institute, 203 Lothrop Street, Pittsburgh, PA 15213, USA; [b] Cranofacial Cleft Surgery, Department of Oral and Maxillofacial Surgery, University of Pittsburgh School of Dental Medicine, 214 Eye and Ear Institute, 203 Lothrop Street, Pittsburgh, PA 15213, USA
* Corresponding author.
E-mail address: bjc1@pitt.edu

Oral Maxillofacial Surg Clin N Am 29 (2017) 9–18
http://dx.doi.org/10.1016/j.coms.2016.08.003

engineering hope to provide custom constructs that become integrated fully in the local anatomy and provide ideal form and function once they are fully integrated into the host. Regenerative medicine can be used to recruit local tissues to produce the desired tissue—ideally in a manner in which the structure and form are useful both aesthetically and functionally.

Three-dimensional scaffolds provide an environment for cells and biomolecules to interact in a specific environment aided by the architectural design of the scaffold.[3] The use of advanced printers for scaffolds has helped overcome challenges in regenerative medicine by enabling the precise positioning of cells and biomaterials in a finely tuned manner.[4] Scaffolds add a welcome layer of complexity to tissue engineering because of the varied styles of 3-dimensional printing and the intricacies of their internal and external architecture.

SOFT TISSUE REGENERATION

Combined techniques of allotransplantation and tissue-engineered constructs has gained some momentum in recent years; rat models in which a rotational latissimus dorsi muscle flap was augmented with in vitro engineered oral mucosa to recreate a functional orbicularis oris complex have been shown.[2] Furthermore, advances have been made in overcoming volumetric deficiency from the loss of fat and muscle. The adipose-derived stem cells are of mesenchymal lineage with characteristic multipotent tendency, which makes their use heterogeneous for not only cell-enriched fat grafting[5] but also restoring volume loss by bony regeneration when coupled with materials such as recombinant human bone morphogenetic protein-2.[6]

The development of tissue-engineered skin has been documented for more than 20 years and has garnered success in the commercial market for grafting and wound repair.[7] Initially, engineered skin was processed neonatal foreskin coupled with bovine type I collagen providing a bilayered skin construct for the use in venous ulcers.[8] Recent techniques have been reported to use mesenchymal stem cells because of their ease of harvest from many sources (bone marrow, adipose tissue, umbilical cord blood, dermis); their inhibitory properties of the inflammatory process; and their ability to synthesize tissue with higher amounts of growth factors, collagen, and angiogenic factors than native fibroblasts.[9]

Advances have also been made in engineering oral tissue constructs by isolating oral fibroblasts and transfecting the cells with a viral carrier to deliver transcription factors to reprogram the cellular microenvironment to create tissues such as mucosa, dental pulp, and oral hard tissues.[10] Tissues engineered or processed that are used as oral mucosa are steadily becoming commercially available with products such as ex vivo–produced oral mucosa equivalent EVPOME and AlloDerm (LifeCell, NJ).[11] Furthermore, the development of highly specialized scaffolds with various cellular and biomolecular approaches has aided in the development of oral tissues such as salivary glands[11] and pulpodentin complexes in a sophisticated and elegant manner.[12]

GROWTH FACTORS IN SOFT TISSUE ENGINEERING

Much of what is known about growth factors in clinical soft tissue engineering comes from studies on platelet-rich plasma (PRP). PRP is a common approach to tissue regeneration strategies in the craniomaxillofacial surgery practice for general improvement of soft and hard tissue healing in the postoperative period.[13] Multiple clinical investigators describe sequestering and concentrating autologous platelets in plasma to serve in surgical sites as grafts to bolster healing responses by the work of primarily 3 growth factors: platelet-derived growth factor (PDGF), transforming growth factor $\beta1$ (TGF-$\beta1$), and transforming growth factor $\beta2$ (TGF-$\beta2$).[14] An initial study by Marx and colleagues[14] on bone regeneration focused on describing the potential clinical use and biologic nature of PDGF and TGF-β growth factors. PDGF is a glycoprotein that is secreted by degranulating platelets and endothelial cells that, in turn, activate cell membrane receptors on target cells that subsequently induce mitogenesis, angiogenesis, and macrophage activation. TGF-β is part of the same superfamily as bone morphogenic protein—they are proteins synthesized by platelets and macrophages and secreted in paracrine fashion to exert effects on neighboring fibroblasts, marrow stem cells, and preosteoblasts.[14] Marx[15] later made the case that PRP may have many clinical uses including not only bone augmentation but also in the preparation and treatment of split-thickness skin grafts (**Fig. 1**).[15] Despite the initial enthusiasm, harnessing the use of this technique has been difficult and this technique has not proven effective in follow-up studies for bone or soft tissue regeneration in a predictable and repeatable way.

PRP has also been used as an adjunct in autologous fat grafting. Liao and colleagues[16] state that although fat grafting aids in reestablishing volumetric soft tissue deficiency, its use is often marred by a 40% to 60% reabsorption rate and

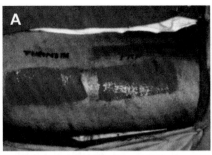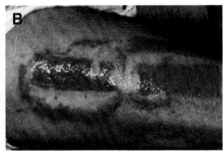

Fig. 1. (*A*) Split-thickness skin graft donor sites at 0.016 inch in depth comparing a control site with a platelet-rich plasma-treated site at the time of initial placement. Note the old skin graft donor site above the platelet-rich plasma-treated site is scarred, contracted, and hyperpigmented. (*B*) The same split-thickness skin graft donor sites as seen in **Fig. 1**A now at 6 days. The control site has a peripheral erythema and is covered by granulation tissue. There is minimal epithelialization. The platelet-rich plasma-treated site has no peripheral erythema. The granulation tissue has already been replaced by a thin epithelial cover at this early stage. (*From* Marx RE. Platelet-rich plasma: evidence to support its use. J Oral Maxillofac Surg 2004;62(4):493; with permission.)

fat necrosis. The use of PRP may help fat graft survival by providing nutrient support from its plasma component, increasing angiogenesis, and enhancing the adipogenic differentiation in the regeneration zone.[16]

Injecting PRP into sites of soft tissue injury, such as muscle or ligament, is documented in the orthopedic literature, and it is used commonly in professional and amateur sports medicine. The healing cascade includes hemostasis followed by inflammation, matrix proliferation, and wound remodeling. Clinically, these techniques have yet to be convincingly proven as effective via level I evidence. The belief is that the use of PRP augments the final phase of wound remodeling by virtue of growth factors PDGF and TGF-β by stimulating fibroblast proliferation and migration for ultimately replacing type III collagen, proteoglycan, and fibronectin for type I collagen for increased tensile strength.[17]

Overall, although PRP has been known anecdotally to have promising results, predictability and reliability based on clinical outcome studies use is less apparent. Based on results from a study performed by Weibrich and colleagues[18] in which growth factors from PRP were isolated using discontinuous cell separation from 115 individuals, the results are largely unpredictable. The study showed "substantial variation" in the resulting concentrations of TGF-β and PDGF.[18] It is probable that PRP has a "shotgun" effect with respect to the release of growth factors, with no predictable, reproducible kinetics, and bioavailability that would be expected of the common scaffold or biologic system, today.[19,20] As such, it may be one of the first steps in producing a more elegant delivery of factors and creating more of a biomimetic environment or delivery system to enhance regeneration and healing.

CELLULAR APPROACHES
Fibroblasts

Cellular approaches in craniomaxillofacial soft tissue regeneration can be broadly discussed for skin regeneration and oral mucosa regeneration. The engineering of skin substitutes for restoring function has been well studied and matured in form to include dermal and mesenchymal support components.[21] Cellular approaches to skin engineering have used various fibroblast phenotypes and genotypes that are different between body sites by their growth kinetics, TGF-β receptor II expression, and mitotic capabilities between superficial and deep dermis layers to name a few. These differences have various implications on the wound healing process.[21] Fibroblasts can also be derived from various pluripotent cell lineages including adult somatic cells, which are reprogramed through the use of various transcription factors that results in cells regaining their ability to transition to another cell line.[22] Different tissues and sizes of defects require various and separate interactions of cells, molecules, matrices, and scaffolds.[3] The goal of engineering is to harness fibroblasts and cultivate them in a milieu that promotes crosstalk with mesenchymal-epidermal growth factors, which, in turn, stimulate keratinocyte proliferation and migration.[21] After induced pluripotent stem cells are differentiated into cell lines like fibroblasts or keratinocytes, they can be engineered in a microenvironment with the aid of a scaffold that can expedite host integration.[10] For instance, dermal constructs have been made with collagen and synthetic polymer scaffolds with seeded biological matrices in an effort to create mesenchymal-epidermal interaction.[21]

Oral Mucosa

Advances have also been made in the develop-ment of oral mucosa from autologous cells in lieu of split-thickness skin grafts. Split-thickness grafts are used ubiquitously for defects; however, they contain adnexal structures and express different patterns of keratinization that vary from normal function of the oral cavity.[22] EVPOME is engineered by procuring autogenous keratinized oral mucosa and seeding onto various dermis scaffolding, such as AlloDerm, and has been used to help close defects including periodontal defects, tumor, and trauma sites.[23] The benefit of using autologous cell lines is the ability to form a construct without immune suppression or rejection.[2] The key to this process is the ability for autologous keratinocytes to seed in the dermal construct, and by reaching critical numbers, constructs are able to mature and differentiate with host tissue beds.[23] The use of EVPOME showed a similar healing pattern to free gingival grafts with successful growth of ker-atinized gingival widths at recipient sites.[24] Ad-vances have been made in rodent models in which EVPOME was combined with latissimus dorsi muscle to create a musculocutaneous flap for use as a rotational or free tissue transfer to recreate the oral opening with functioning musculature.[2]

Bony support for soft tissue such as oral mu-cosa has been reported with the use of either autogenous flaps or scaffolds.[25] Microvascular fibula flaps have been either prelaminated with oral mucosa constructs before inset into a defect or covered with autologous keratinized oral mu-cosa in a second stage after inset, with both

showing successful results with dental implant placement.[25]

A study looking at biodegradable scaffolds as car-riers for autologous oral mucosa including polylac-tide meshes, tendon collagen-glycosaminoglycan constructs, and collagen membranes (**Fig. 2**) found all 3 to result in epithelial morphology of fibroblast ingrowth and keratinocyte speciation but with various differences in tissue thickness and robust-ness of fibroblast ingrowth. Vicryl mesh showed lack of significant fibroblast migration into the scaffold because of the mesh structure, whereas ingrowth was successful in the collagen-based scaffolds.[26] Another study used a collagen-glycosaminoglycan-chitosan scaffold with fibro-blasts, which resulted in the development of a lamina propria equivalent and an oral mucosa equiv-alent.[27] The combination of these cellular ap-proaches in a sophisticated scaffold construct holds promise for the more efficient and predictable closure of facial defects.

SCAFFOLDS

Scaffolds are implantable or injectable constructs engineered for the delivery of cells and proteins to create a favorable environment for cell attach-ment, proliferation, differentiation of function, and migration.[28] Scaffolds have been used success-fully in various fields of tissue engineering including bone formation, periodontal regenera-tion, cartilage construction, corneas, heart valves, and tendons.[28] Scaffolds serve as a reservoir of nutrients for microenvironments and macroenvir-onments and as a structural support system for tissue growth; in the context of craniofacial

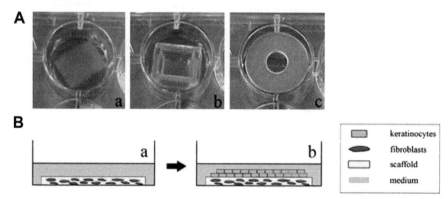

Fig. 2. Culture system: (*A*) (a) 1- × 1.3-cm piece of scaffold in 1 well of a 12-well plate, (b) fixation of the scaffold with a polystyrene frame to assure that cells grow on the epidermal side of the scaffold, (c) stabilization with a titanium ring to avoid shifting of the frame. (*B*) (a) Dermal equivalent (DE): fibroblasts grown in the scaffold, (b) oral mucosa equivalent: keratinocytes grown on the DE. (*From* Kriegebaum U, Mildenberger M, Mueller-Richter UD, et al. Tissue engineering of human oral mucosa on different scaffolds: in vitro experiments as a basis for clin-ical applications. Oral Surg Oral Med Oral Pathol Oral Radiol 2012;114(5 Suppl):S192; with permission.)

engineering, the scaffold is a transitory template that helps the development of the extracellular matrix in the support of both hard and soft tissue regeneration and maturation.[3]

The construct of a scaffold has become highly specialized with respect to the type of tissue being developed. Despite this specialization, the fundamental properties shared by all intricately engineered 3-dimensional scaffold architectures are porosity, interconnectivity, and the mechanical integrity by which they are upheld in vivo.[29] To maintain the intrinsic biocompatibility in an in vivo environment, the biological cross talk between cells must be controlled by the properties of the scaffold; its mechanical properties and degradation kinetics are influenced by the porosity, surface area exposure, and penetrance of cells within the scaffold volume to allow for an effective regenerative process.[30]

Scaffolds allow for the delivery of progenitor cells and growth factors while maintaining an architecture that is congruent with the defect the scaffold is obturating.[31] The types of scaffolds and properties necessary by each for bone engineering have been well established[3,31]; however, scaffolds for soft tissue engineering have not shared the same uniform study in part because of the broad range of soft tissue that has been engineered in the fields of cardiac, neurologic, and orthopedic regeneration.[32,33] Attempts at using autologous cells from pulpal or gingival fibroblasts compounded with polymer scaffolds such as polyglycolic acid (PGA) have been described; however, success has been limited because of the inherent disadvantages of polymers such as the acidification of the environment on dissolution[34] and difficulty in reproducing successful rates of cell-seeding in the construct.[35]

Collagen scaffolds have been used broadly for the reconstruction of various soft tissues in craniomaxillofacial regeneration.[36] Collagen is an abundant protein, and its biocompatibility and support of angiogenesis makes it a common source for scaffold construction. Collagen's benefit with respect to oral tissue regeneration has been that its intrinsic properties led to immediate wound healing when obturated in the defect with the release of PDGF, which triggers the repair process.[36] Current limitations of collagen scaffolds are that the intrinsic properties of the protein make its degradation highly variable and attempts at slowing degradation by cross-linking induces a foreign body reaction.[36] The use of *chitosan* as a vehicle in the scaffold construct has led for greater predictive release of factors such as PDGF by platelets; this has also enhanced the proliferation and differentiation of stem cells.[37] Chitosan, which

is a deacetylated derivative of chitin, possesses drug-delivery and antimicrobial properties in addition to the aforementioned proliferative and wound healing properties, which has garnered accelerated use in periodontal regeneration and the construction of ligaments, blood vessels, skin, mucosa, and musculofascia when the chitosan scaffold is compounded with the proper cellular system.[38] Chitosan scaffold constructs have even been found to enhance the effects of PRP, which is highly inconsistent by itself, with respect to regulating the release kinetics of growth factors such as insulinlike growth factor-1 and PDGF.[39]

Engineering of musculotendinous constructs also uses the natural process of wound healing by hastening the repair process of myoblast migration and differentiation by creating specialized macrophage-based scaffolds.[40] The key feature of musculotendinous regeneration has been overcoming volumetric muscle loss after surgical procedures such as tumor extirpation or trauma.[41] To rebulk these defects, the myofiber and components of the basement membrane such as the type IV collagen, glycosaminoglycans, proteoglycans, laminins, and fibronectin need to be replicated; the use of various scaffolds including synthetic polymers such as PGA and natural polymers such as alginate, collagen, and fibrin increase the survival of implanted cell constructs.[32] Although success has been seen in the development of transplantable tissues including skin, cartilage, and bone, issues remain with respect to challenges in high-resolution cell deposition, controlled cell distribution, vascularization, and innervation within the tissue.[42]

THREE-DIMENSIONAL CONSTRUCTS IN TISSUE ENGINEERING

A 3-dimensional scaffold has a sophisticated design that allows for not only a bioresorbable platform as seen in synthetics like PGA, but also a bioactive nature that augments the ability of implanted cells and constructs to grow in a defect site, particularly with respect to maintaining volume and tissue bulk, a constant problem in soft tissue engineering.[43] Conventional tissue engineering approaches have not been able to seed cells in a scaffold in a uniform distribution with placement of cells and growth factors, nor has it been able to predictably create a vascular system that can support a thick or complex tissue.[44] The goals for 3-dimensional biomanufactured scaffolds are to develop craniofacial tissue analogs in which all components that form a tissue, cells, and matrix materials, can be printed in a precise manner using computer-aided design (CAD) software and 3-dimensional imaging modality such as computed tomography.[4]

Computer-Aided Design and Computer-Aided Manufacturing

CAD and computer-aided manufacturing (CAD/CAM) with 3-dimensional printing has been in use for some time in dentistry and medicine for fabrication of various dental and medical materials such as titanium implants and restorative crowns. With respect to soft tissue regeneration, biomimetic scaffolds made of polycaprolactone impregnated with chondrogenic growth factors in a hyaluronic acid/collagen hydrogel have been designed using CAD/CAM and printed for use in nasal and auricular reconstruction.[45] CAD/CAM procedures used for computer-assisted surgery typically involve 3 steps: (1) virtual planning by obtaining Digital Imaging and Communications in Medicine (DICOM) images that are transferred as a stereolithographic file to a CAD program, (2) manufacturing of the custom-made scaffold using a milling machine that produces the shape and specifications of the CAD, (3) reconstructive surgery for inset of the construct.[46] The use of these strategies in pediatric populations with microtia has been shown using collagen type I hydrogel scaffolds that were of high fidelity and biocompatibility in contrast to dated techniques of costal cartilage grafting. Geometric complexities of scaffold constructs were printed after using 3-dimensional computed tomography imaging or photogrammetry that were processed using CAD/CAM software to ultimately print a mold from which implants were fabricated in an intricate manner using various biomimetic materials and factors.[47]

Scaffold Printing

Three-dimensional scaffolds can be made by inkjet printing, laser-assisted printing, or extrusion printing. Extrusion printing has been used commonly in the production of hard tissue constructs in craniomaxillofacial surgery.[48] Inkjet printing is the most prolific process to form constructs in soft tissue engineering and is defined as a noncontact printing technique that reproduces digital pattern information onto a substrate with tiny ink drops.[44] "Bioink" is matrix material that is used for inkjet printing and is central to generating a large-volume 3-dimensional structure that can provide cues and signals for cell function and tissue formation.[49] The extracellular matrix for soft tissue provides constant physical, chemical, and biological support for the structural components necessary for collagen and fibrin growth

during healing and regeneration.[49] The bioink can be placed by thermal, piezoelectric, or electromagnetic approaches, each with a rather nuanced means of meticulously placing the ink onto a construct.[44] For instance, in thermal printing, the temperature gradient, frequency of current, pulse, and predetermined ink viscosity help provide the release of pressurized air bubbles to inject ink drops of volumes ranging from 10 to 150 pL.[44] With respect to craniofacial engineering, hard and soft tissue regeneration can be accomplished by combining the appropriate growth factors and cell lines and coupling them with a scaffold specific for the desired tissue to be replicated, including polymer hydrogels, ceramics, and inert metals.[4] Recently, the goals of 3-dimensional printing have been to place living mammalian cells on scaffold or scaffoldless aggregates to form hard and soft tissues[4,44]; however, the challenge with the placement of living cells has been to avoid cell lysis and heat damage from current inkjet printing techniques. This is not limited to inkjet printing, but also seen with laser-assisted printing despite its ability to provide various viscosities of bioink not seen in inkjet printing.[4]

Recently, 3-dimensional bioprinting was used to develop skin by using human dermal fibroblasts and an electromagnetic inkjet technology by alternating layers of fibroblasts with extracellular matrix component bioink in a precise manner using cell-compatible printheads that would limit the issues seen elsewhere with viscosity, cell lysis, and damage.[50]

The use of CAD/CAM-developed scaffolds with bone marrow stromal cell sheets was recently demonstrated to successfully develop periosteumlike tissue that has promise to accelerate healing in defect sites (**Fig. 3**).[51] The creation of these 3-dimensional calcium phosphate scaffolds using inkjet printing was thus able to exhibit the desired biofunctional attributes of biocompatibility, bioactivity, safety, and internal and external microstructure and macrostructure combined with the desired spatial and temporal pharmacokinetic transport response when coupled with cell sheets that were designed with the intent of creating periosteum and bonelike tissue (**Figs. 4 and 5**).[3]

VASCULAR REGENERATION

One of the most intriguing aspects of tissue engineering has been the challenge of encouraging neovascularization—particularly for large defects. Although it has become quite straightforward to provide a large mass of cells to a defect in a given scaffold, providing adequate blood supply to

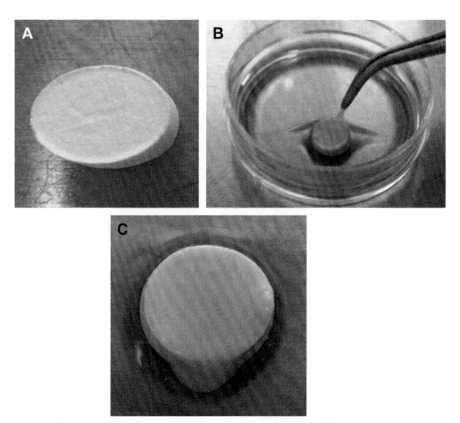

Fig. 3. Images of calcium phosphate (*A*) before being wrapped with the cell sheet and (*B*) as it is being wrapped with the cell sheet. (*C*) The calcium phosphate scaffold with the cell sheet wrap before implantation. (*From* Syed-Picard FN, Shah GA, Costello BJ, et al. Regeneration of periosteum by human bone marrow stromal cell sheets. J Oral Maxillofac Surg 2014;72(6):1080; with permission.)

sustain those cells throughout the graft has proven difficult. Additionally, providing a conduit for application of growth factors within a wound for temporal release throughout the regenerative process has also been challenging. Many approaches have been considered to address these concerns. Much is understood about the process of normal vascular development, neoangiogenesis in the

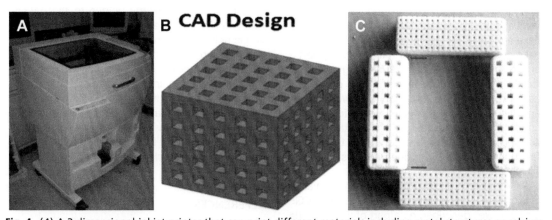

Fig. 4. (*A*) A 3-dimensional inkjet printer that can print different materials including metal structures or calcium phosphate cement material from standard imaging software. (*B*) Digital Imaging and Communications in Medicine (DICOM) images can be imported into the software, where the scaffolding can be adjusted and redesigned for printing. (*C*) Custom constructs can be printed for use with proteins, cells, or other materials for regenerating tissues. (*From* Costello BJ, Shah G, Kumta P, et al. Regenerative medicine for craniomaxillofacial surgery. Oral Maxillofac Surg Clin North Am 2010;22(1):37; with permission.)

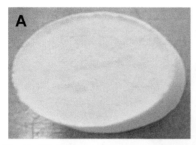 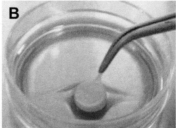 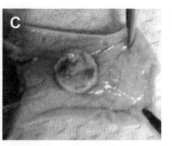

Fig. 5. (*A*) Calcium phosphate before manipulation with cells. (*B*) Calcium phosphate being enveloped with a cell sheet. (*C*) Calcium phosphate scaffold with a cell sheet wrap after explantation showing invagination of cell lines over the scaffold construct. (*From* Costello BJ, Shah G, Kumta P, et al. Regenerative medicine for craniomaxillofacial surgery. Oral Maxillofac Surg Clin North Am 2010;22(1):33–42; with permission.)

adult, and the genes that are involved in vascular development as well.[52,53] There is a complex dynamic that occurs during vascular development including extrinsic influences, flow physics, hypoxia, and other factors.[54,55] Many scientists working in this area believe that once the issue of vascular regeneration is adequately addressed, it will open a door of opportunity not yet seen for regenerative medicine.

The process of neovascularization involves the interaction of endothelial cells and their formation of a primitive blood vessel plexus, which becomes a network of arteries, veins, and their associated capillaries. This process is thought to be tightly regulated with various signal pathways and involves the interaction of the local environment and the regulation of genes important in vascular development. The vascular endothelial growth factors (VEGFs) involved in this process are thought to drive this system forward in the proper manner. As such, the simple deposition of one particular type of VEGF at a high concentration within a wound is not likely to reproduce a complex vasculature system. The temporal release of these and other factors in the proper environment make creating a vasculature that could support a regenerative tissue construct challenging. Additionally, there are several pathologic processes that likely involve inappropriate VEGF upregulation such as arteriovascular malformations, tumor growth, and aneurysm formation. Understanding this complex mechanism is the key to developing a tissue-engineered construct that will have appropriate vascular support.

VEGF appears to have a key role in the tissue development and regenerative processes. VEGF has been well described as a part of the cascade controlling bone development during the promotion of vascular structures, particularly in the process of bone healing by acting on bone-forming cells.[53,56,57] Taking advantage of this growth factor is more challenging than just delivering it to a site with the expectation that vascular tissues will regenerate. There are dose effect concerns as well as the importance of the temporal release of factors during a healing/regeneration phase that is appropriate. Kaigler and colleagues[58] reported some interesting work in this area, including the use of a VEGF-based scaffold that showed improved neovascularization and bone regeneration in a critical size rat calvarial defect exposed to radiation.

SUMMARY

Regenerative medicine has impacted craniomaxillofacial surgery in both hard and soft tissue reconstruction. Today, the merging of technologies using existing knowledge of scaffolds, cellular pathways, and CAD/CAM software enables clinicians and scientists to enjoy new ventures in regeneration of tissue by elegant design. The continued efforts with novel materials give way to produce 3-dimensional tissue constructs that are biocompatible and nearly unique to the patient. Additionally, our understanding of neovascularization is helping tailor our approaches to soft tissue regeneration. By combining our understanding of signaling molecules, scaffolds, and cellular technology, and designing 3-dimensional constructs through the through the use of various biometric printers, we can expand the regenerative possibilities seen in various animal and human models. Surgeons who work in the craniomaxillofacial region must have a clear understanding of these concepts.

REFERENCES

1. Susarla SM, Swanson E, Gordon CR. Craniomaxillofacial reconstruction using allotransplantation and tissue engineering: challenges, opportunities, and potential synergy. Ann Plast Surg 2011;67(6): 655–61.

2. Kim RY, Fasi AC, Feinberg SE. Soft tissue engineering in craniomaxillofacial surgery. Ann Maxillofac Surg 2014;4(1):4–8.
3. Costello BJ, Shah G, Kumta P, et al. Regenerative medicine for craniomaxillofacial surgery. Oral Maxillofac Surg Clin North Am 2010;22(1):33–42.
4. Obregon F, Vaquette C, Ivanovski S, et al. Three-dimensional bioprinting for regenerative dentistry and craniofacial tissue engineering. J Dent Res 2015;94(Suppl 9):143S–52S.
5. Minteer DM, Marra KG, Rubin JP. Adipose stem cells: biology, safety, regulation, and regenerative potential. Clin Plast Surg 2015;42(2):169–79.
6. Sandor GK. Tissue engineering of bone: Clinical observations with adipose-derived stem cells, resorbable scaffolds, and growth factors. Ann Maxillofac Surg 2012;2(1):8–11.
7. Bello YM, Falabella AF, Eaglstein WH. Tissue-engineered skin. Current status in wound healing. Am J Clin Dermatol 2001;2(5):305–13.
8. Trent JF, Kirsner RS. Tissue engineered skin: Apligraf, a bi-layered living skin equivalent. Int J Clin Pract 1998;52(6):408–13.
9. Hu MS, Leavitt T, Malhotra S, et al. Stem cell-based therapeutics to improve wound healing. Plast Surg Int 2015;2015:383581.
10. Hewitt KJ, Shamis Y, Gerami-Naini B, et al. Strategies for oral mucosal repair by engineering 3D tissues with pluripotent stem cells. Adv Wound Care (New Rochelle) 2014;3(12):742–50.
11. Rai R, Raval R, Khandeparker RV, et al. Tissue engineering: Step ahead in maxillofacial reconstruction. J Int Oral Health 2015;7(9):138–42.
12. Qu T, Jing J, Ren Y, et al. Complete pulpodentin complex regeneration by modulating the stiffness of biomimetic matrix. Acta Biomater 2015;16:60–70.
13. Albanese A, Licata ME, Polizzi B, et al. Platelet-rich plasma (PRP) in dental and oral surgery: from the wound healing to bone regeneration. Immun Ageing 2013;10(1):23.
14. Marx RE, Carlson ER, Eichstaedt RM, et al. Platelet-rich plasma: Growth factor enhancement for bone grafts. Oral Surg Oral Med Oral Pathol Oral Radiol Endod 1998;85(6):638–46.
15. Marx RE. Platelet-rich plasma: evidence to support its use. J Oral Maxillofac Surg 2004;62(4):489–99.
16. Liao HT, Marra KG, Rubin JP. Application of platelet-rich plasma and platelet-rich fibrin in fat grafting: basic science and literature review. Tissue Eng Part B Rev 2014;20(4):267–76.
17. Middleton KK, Barro V, Muller B, et al. Evaluation of the effects of platelet-rich plasma (PRP) therapy involved in the healing of sports-related soft tissue injuries. Iowa Orthop J 2012;32:150–63.
18. Weibrich G, Kleis WK, Hafner G, et al. Growth factor levels in platelet-rich plasma and correlations with donor age, sex, and platelet count. J Craniomaxillofac Surg 2002;30(2):97–102.
19. Sanchez AR, Sheridan PJ, Kupp LI. Is platelet-rich plasma the perfect enhancement factor? A current review. Int J Oral Maxillofac Implants 2003;18(1):93–103.
20. Tozum TF, Demiralp B. Platelet-rich plasma: a promising innovation in dentistry. J Can Dent Assoc 2003;69(10):664.
21. Nolte SV, Xu W, Rennekampff HO, et al. Diversity of fibroblasts—a review on implications for skin tissue engineering. Cells Tissues Organs 2008;187(3):165–76.
22. Izumi K, Song J, Feinberg SE. Development of tissue-engineered human oral mucosa: from the bench to the bed side. Cells Tissues Organs 2004;176(1–3):134–52.
23. Kato H, Marcelo CL, Washington JB, et al. Fabrication of Large Size Ex-Vivo Produced Oral Mucosal Equivalents for Clinical Application. Tissue Eng Part C Methods 2015;21(9):872–80.
24. Izumi K, Neiva RF, Feinberg SE. Intraoral grafting of tissue-engineered human oral mucosa. Int J Oral Maxillofac Implants 2013;28(5):e295–303.
25. Sieira GR, Pages CM, Diez EG, et al. Tissue-engineered oral mucosa grafts for intraoral lining reconstruction of the maxilla and mandible with fibula flap. J Oral Maxillofac Surg 2015;73(1):195.e1–6.
26. Kriegebaum U, Mildenberger M, Mueller-Richter UD, et al. Tissue engineering of human oral mucosa on different scaffolds: in vitro experiments as a basis for clinical applications. Oral Surg Oral Med Oral Pathol Oral Radiol 2012;114(5 Suppl):S190–8.
27. Kinikoglu B, Auxenfaus C, Pierrillas P, et al. Reconstruction of a full thickness collagen-based human oral mucosal equivalent. Biomaterials 2009;30(32):6418–25.
28. Garg T, Singh O, Arora S, et al. Scaffold: a novel carrier for cell and drug delivery. Crit Rev Ther Drug Carrier Syst 2012;29(1):1–63.
29. Mallick KK, Cox SC. Biomaterial scaffolds for tissue engineering. Front Biosci (Elite Ed) 2013;5:341–60.
30. Carletti E, Endogan T, Hasirci V, et al. Microfabrication of PDLLA scaffolds. J Tissue Eng Regen Med 2011;5(7):669–77.
31. Teven CM, Fisher S, Ameer GA. Biomimetic approaches to complex craniofacial defects. Ann Maxillofac Surg 2015;5(1):4–13.
32. Grasman JM, Zayas MJ, Page RL, et al. Biomimetic scaffolds for regeneration of volumetric muscle loss in skeletal muscle injuries. Acta Biomater 2015;25:2–15.
33. Rosenzweig DH, Carelli E, Steffen T, et al. 3D-printed ABS and PLA Scaffolds for Cartilage and Nucleus Pulposus Tissue Regeneration. Int J Mol Sci 2015;16(7):15118–35.

34. Buurma B, Gu K, Rutherford RB. Transplantation of huma pulpal and gingival fibroblasts attached to synthetic scaffolds. Eur J Oral Sci 1999;107(4): 282–9.

35. Hillmann G, Steinkamp-Zucht A, Geurtsen W, et al. Culture of primary human gingival fibroblasts on biodegradable membranes. Biomaterials 2002; 23(6):1461–9.

36. Agis H, Collins A, Taut AD, et al. Cell population kinetics of collagen scaffolds in ex vivo oral wound repair. PLoS One 2014;9(11):e112680.

37. Busilacchi A, Gigante A, Mattioli-Belmonte M, et al. Chitosan stabilizes platelet growth factors and modulates stem cell differentiation toward tissue regeneration. Carbohydr Polym 2013;98(1):665–76.

38. Silva D, Arancibia R, Tapia C, et al. Chitosan and platelet-derived growth factor synergistically stimulate cell proliferation in gingival fibroblasts. J Periodontal Res 2013;48(6):677–86.

39. Kutlu B, Tigli Aydin RS, Akman AC, et al. Platelet-rich plasma-loaded chitosan scaffolds: preparation and growth factor release kinetics. J Biomed Mater Res B Appl Biomater 2013;101(1):28–35.

40. Turner NJ, Badylak SF. Biologic scaffolds for musculotendinous tissue repair. Eur Cell Mater 2013;25: 130–43.

41. Mertens JP, Sugg KB, Lee JD, et al. Engineering muscle constructs for the creation of functional engineered musculoskeletal tissue. Regen Med 2014; 9(1):89–100.

42. Mandrycky C, Wang Z, Kim K, et al. 3D bioprinting for engineering complex tissues. Biotechnol Adv 2016;34(4):422–34.

43. Zuk PA. Tissue engineering craniofacial defects with adult stem cells? Are we ready yet? Pediatr Res 2008;63(5):478–86.

44. Cui X, Boland T, D'Lima DD, et al. Thermal inkjet printing in tissue engineering and regenerative medicine. Recent Pat Drug Deliv Formul 2012; 6(2):149–55.

45. Zopf DA, Mitsak AG, Flanagan CL, et al. Computer aided-designed, 3-dimensionally printed porous tissue bioscaffolds for craniofacial soft tissue reconstruction. Otolaryngol Head Neck Surg 2015; 152(1):57–62.

46. Mangano F, Macchi A, Shibli JA, et al. Maxillary ridge augmentation with custom-made CAD/CAM scaffolds. A 1-year prospective study on 10 patients. J Oral Implantol 2014;40(5):561–9.

47. Reiffel AJ, Kafka C, Hernandez KA, et al. High-fidelity tissue engineering of patient-specific auricles for reconstruction of pediatric microtia and other auricular deformities. PLoS One 2013;8(2): e56506.

48. Hollister SJ. Porous scaffold design for tissue engineering. Nat Mater 2005;4(7):518–24.

49. Pati F, Ha DH, Jang J, et al. Biomimetic 3D tissue printing for soft tissue regeneration. Biomaterials 2015;62:164–75.

50. Rimann M, Bono E, Annaheim H, et al. Standardized 3D Bioprinting of soft tissue models with human primary cells. J Lab Autom 2015;21(4):496–509.

51. Syed-Picard FN, Shah GA, Costello BJ, et al. Regeneration of periosteum by human bone marrow stromal cell sheets. J Oral Maxillofac Surg 2014;72(6): 1078–83.

52. Carmeliet P. Angiogenesis in health and disease. Nat Med 2003;9:653–60.

53. Coultas L, Chawengsaksophak K, Rossant J. Endothelial cells and VEGF in vascular development. Nature 2005;438:937–45.

54. Ramirez-Bergeron A, Runge K, Dahl HJ, et al. Hypoxia affects mesoderm and enhances hemangioblast specification during early development. Development 2003;130:4393–403.

55. Le Noble F, Moyan D, Pardanaud L, et al. Flow regulates arterial-venous differentiation in the chick embryo yolk sac. Development 2004;131:361–75.

56. Street J, Bao M, deGuzman L, et al. Vascular endothelial growth factor stimulates bone repair by promoting angiogenesis and bone turnover. Proc Natl Acad Sci U S A 2002;99:9656–61.

57. Nakagawa M, Kaneda T, Arakawa T, et al. Vascular endothelial growth factor (VEGF) directly enhances osteoclastic bone resorption and survival of mature osteoclasts. FEBS Lett 2000;473:161–4.

58. Kaigler D, Wang Z, Horger K, et al. VEGF scaffolds enhance angiogenesis and bone regeneration in irradiated osseous defects. J Bone Miner Res 2006;21:735–43.

Applications of Mesenchymal Stem Cells in Oral and Craniofacial Regeneration

Pasha Shakoori, DDS, MA, Quanzhou Zhang, PhD,
Anh D. Le, DDS, PhD*

KEYWORDS

- Stem cells • Orofacial mesenchymal stem cells • Regenerative medicine • Tissue engineering

KEY POINTS

- The field of tissue engineering and regenerative medicine has been rapidly expanded through multidisciplinary integration of research and clinical practice in response to the unmet clinical needs for reconstruction of the dental, oral, and craniofacial structures.
- The significance of the various types of stem cells, specifically mesenchymal stem cells (MSCs) derived from the orofacial tissues, ranging from dental pulp stem cells (DPSCs) to periodontal ligament stem cells (PDLSCs) to mucosa/gingiva (gingiva-derived MSCs [GMSCs]) has been thoroughly investigated.
- Currently, there are several clinical trials aimed to further study the applications of oral and craniofacial stem cells in regeneration.

INTRODUCTION

Reconstruction of oral and craniofacial defects has been a challenging task for many clinicians. Since McGregor performed the first flap (temporalis) in the reconstruction of a postexcisional defect in the oral cavity in 1963,[1] many clinicians have attempted to modify surgical techniques in flap transfer to improve the functional outcomes. In many cases, however, complete restoration of the original anatomy and function is not possible regardless of the surgical technique used. This problem is further evident in the oral and craniofacial region considering the importance of functions, such as speech, mastication, appearance, and the effects of these deficiencies on general health, social acceptance, and self-esteem.[2]

Considering the limitations of reconstructive techniques, regenerative medicine and tissue engineering have been new avenues explored by scientists and clinicians to restore anatomy and function. In simplified terms, to regenerate tissue, a source of stem cells, a 3-D platform (scaffold), and a source of signaling molecules are needed.

The classic definition of a stem cell requires such cells to have 2 fundamental characteristics: self-renewal and potency. Allowing for self-renewal requires the capacity of a cell to divide without differentiation; potency specifies the capacity to differentiate into different cell types.

The authors have nothing to disclose.
Funded by: NIH; Grant number: NIH/NIDCR R01 DE019932, Osteo Science Foundation, Oral & Maxillofacial Surgery Foundation (OMSF) Research Grant.
Department of Oral and Maxillofacial Surgery/Pharmacology, University of Pennsylvania, School of Dental Medicine, 240 South 40th Street, Philadelphia, PA 19104-6030, USA
* Corresponding author.
E-mail address: Anh.Le@uphs.upenn.edu

Table 1
Orofacial stem cells and clinical applications

MSCs	Markers	Animal Models	Studies	Disease Models
PDLSC	STRO-1, CD146/MUC18	Mouse	Seo et al,[22] 2004	
		Swine	Liu et al,[23] 2008	Periodontitis
		Swine	Ding et al,[24] 2010	Periodontitis
DPSC	CD105+	Dog	Kerkis et al,[42] 2008	Muscular dystrophy
		Rat	Gandia et al,[43] 2008	Myocardial infarct
		Rabbit	Monteiro et al,[44] 2009	Cerebral ischemia
		Rabbit	Gomes et al,[45] 2010	Chemical-induced corneal injury
SHED	Oct-4, Nanog, SSEA-3, SSEA-4, TRA-1-60, TRA-1-81	Rat	Wang et al,[46] 2010	Parkinson disease
GMSC	Oct-4, SSEA-4, STRO-1	Mouse	Zhang et al,[33] 2009	Colitis
		Mouse	Zhang et al,[32] 2010	Wound healing
		Mouse	Su et al,[35] 2011	Contact hypersensitivity
		Rat	Wang, 2011[47]	Mandibular and calvarial defects
		Rat	Zhang et al,[48] 2013	Arthritis
SCAP	STRO-1	Swine	Sonoyama et al,[21] 2006	Tooth regeneration

There are 3 categories of stem cells: adult stem cells (ASCs), embryonic stem cells, and induced pluripotent stem cells (iPSCs). MSCs, which are found in many tissue sources, such as bone marrow and periosteum, are undifferentiated ASCs that are clonogenic and have the capacity to self-renew and differentiate into different cell lines. In vitro expansion of MSC results in cells that are fibroblast-like morphologically and can differentiate into osteoblasts, chondrocytes, adipocytes, and other cells.[3] Although embryonic stem cells are found only in the blastocyst stage of development, ASCs can be found in many adult tissues, in addition to bone marrow and periosteum, including the orofacial tissues (**Table 1**), such as teeth, dental pulp, supporting structures, and gingiva as well as fat, muscle, nervous tissues, skin, and others. iPSCs, a new source of pluripotent stem cells, can be derived from adult cells by introducing 4 pluripotency genes (Oct4, Sox2, cMyc, and Klf4), which are also called Yamanaka factors, named after Shinya Yamanaka, who was the first to generate iPSCs and later awarded the Nobel Prize in Physiology or Medicine in 2012 along with John B. Gurdon for this discovery.[3]

BONE MARROW MESENCHYMAL STEM CELLS IN ORAL AND CRANIOFACIAL REGENERATION

Considering the nature and extent of structural defects in oral and maxillofacial region, many investigators have aimed to regenerate bone, cartilage, and fat using adult BMSCs. This advancement further resulted in attempts to create composite structures made of different tissue types. For instance, the condylar head of the temporomandibular joint complex contains a cartilaginous articular component housed over subchondral bone. In a study performed by Alhadlaq and colleagues,[4] the investigators induced rat BMSCs into osteogenic and chondrogenic cell lineages in vitro. The osteogenic and chondrogenic cells were further incorporated in polyethylene glycol–based hydrogel suspensions in 2 distinct and parallel hydrogel layers, which were sequentially photopolymerized in a human condylar mold. This cell-polymer solution resulted in the formation of cross-links in the mold that created the stratified organization of the bone and cartilage layers of the condylar head. This engineered condyle head was then transplanted into the dorsum of mice for 8 weeks and when harvested demonstrated stratified layers of bone and cartilage cells. The results of this study were further supported by the histologic and immunohistological studies and further expression profiles of these 2 distinct cell types. The results of this study can be considered primitive proof of the concept regarding the potential to use tissue engineering to create and replace composite structural components in the oral and maxillofacial region using adult BMSCs. Using a different approach, other researchers have used a gradient scaffold with incorporated bone morphogenetic protein 2 on the osteogenic side and transforming growth factor-β1 on the chondrogenic side to repair composite osteo-chondral defects.[5]

MESENCHYMAL STEM CELLS DERIVED FROM OROFACIAL TISSUES

Compared with BMSCs isolated from long bones, BMSCs isolated from craniofacial bones show different characteristics and gene expression profile.[6] This difference is mostly attributed to most craniofacial bones arising from neural crest cells[7,8]; hence, many congenital bone diseases, such as Treacher-Collins syndrome,[9] craniofacial fibrous dysplasia,[10] and cherubism,[11] only affect the craniofacial bones, despite that the genes involved in causing the anomalies are expressed in other bones in the body as well. Notably, the craniofacial BMSCs proliferate faster, have increased levels of alkaline phosphatase, and form higher levels of compact bone compared with long bone BMSCs.[12,13] It has been proposed that the progenitor cells responsible for repair of craniofacial bony structures after injury reside in the craniofacial periosteum.[14] In addition to cells residing in the periosteum, craniofacial sutures contain specific MSCs called *Gli1+*, which are quiescent stem cells capable of regenerating dura and periosteum tissue once activated after sustaining injuries.[15] Identification of these cells might further clarify the mechanism of development of craniosynostosis considering that destruction of *Gli1+* cells in open cranial sutures results in premature closure of sutures.[15]

Mesenchymal Stem Cells Derived from Dental Pulps

Other efforts to identify new sources of MSCs have resulted in the isolation of stem cells from different orofacial regions. Postnatal human DPSCs have the potential to regenerate dentin/pulplike complexes and are hypothesized to be the progenitor cells activated when the pulp complex is in need of repair. Previously, studies had shown the odontogenic potential of dental pulp by showing mineralizing capacity using techniques such as cell-culture explants.[16–19] New studies show, however, that DPSCs show many specific similarities compared with BMSCs. These 2 populations of stem cells are both clonogenic, are highly proliferative, and have the capacity to regenerate tissue. The immune-histochemical analyses of human DPSCs and BMSCs in vitro have shown similar immunoreactivity profiles for both groups of cells. Furthermore, both groups of cells express endothelial and smooth muscle cell markers.[20] On the other hand, BMSCs are capable of forming lamellar bone when transplanted into mice, whereas transplanted DPSCs form odontoblast-like cells capable of forming dentin-like complexes under the same conditions.[7]

DPSCs have been used to create bio-engineered dental root (bioroot complex) in swine (**Fig. 1**).[21] Investigators were able to create a bioengineered root complex in swine by using autologous DPSCs, scaffold constructs composed of tricalcium phosphate and hydroxyapatite, and appropriate growth factors with proper tissue conditions. A biological scaffold is a 3-D construct that can be impregnated with different growth factors, such as bone morphogenic protein, that provide the 3-D morphology required for the deposition of an extracellular matrix, which provides a better environment for cell adhesion and migration in regeneration. Such scaffolds can be created with materials that are incorporated into the engineered structure, such as hydroxyapatite or materials that resorb and only leave the newly generated structure. The created bioroot in this study was then harvested after 6 months and implanted in an extraction socket that was artificially created in the swine jaw bone and was later restored using a crown. This study illustrates the potential of creating a biological root complex using DPSCs under the appropriate conditions and use of the correct scaffolds.

Mesenchymal Stem Cells Derived from Periodontal Ligaments

Periodontal ligament tissues have also shown to house PDLSCs. Once cultured in appropriate conditions, PDLSCs are capable of differentiating into cementoblast-like cells, adipocytes, and cells with the capacity to form collagen.[22]

Autologous transplantation of PDLSCs in a miniature porcine model of periodontitis has been shown effective in treating periodontal disease, resulting in regeneration of periodontal tissue in a surgically created periodontal defect (see **Fig. 1**).[23] Moreover, considering the limitations in using autologous cells, especially in older population of patients, allogeneic PDLSCs have been used to treat bone and periodontal defects.[24] Periodontal disease, in addition to compromising oral and dental tissue, has been associated with a variety of systemic conditions, such as cardiovascular disease and diabetes,[25] and the application of these cells in treating periodontitis could have a significant impact in improving oral and systemic health in the general population and result in a reduction of health care costs.

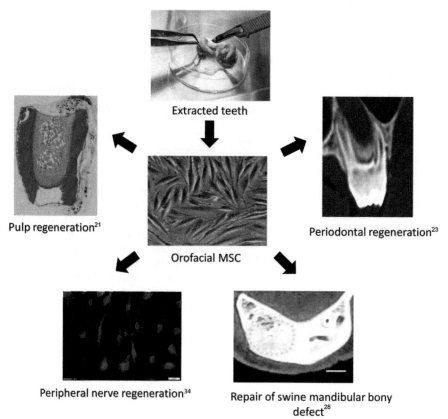

Fig. 1. Regeneration of the dental, oral, and craniofacial tissues using orofacial MSCs. (*From* Refs.[21,23,28,34]; with permission.)

Mesenchymal Stem Cells Derived from Developing Teeth

Vascularized tissues of dental pulp in addition to dentin have been regenerated using 2 other sources of stem cells from the oral cavity: stem cells from apical papilla (SCAP) and stem cells from human exfoliated deciduous teeth (SHED).[24–27] SCAP and other types of pulp stem cells have potentials for pulp/dentin regeneration, and the combination of SCAP and PDLSCs for bioroot engineering has been reported by Sonoyama and colleagues[21] (see **Fig. 1**). Orofacial MSCs have also shown the potential and capacity to regenerate bone in larger defects. SHED-mediated jaw bone regeneration in miniature swine[28] demonstrated the potential of stem cell applications in regeneration of large defects in larger animal models, which could lead to the conduction of human clinical trials aiming to regenerate and repair mandibular bony defects (see **Fig. 1**). For instance, investigators have used MSC implantation in treatment of osteonecrosis of the jaw in swine.[29]

Sinus augmentation and repair of alveolar bone defects have been major tasks in oral and maxillofacial rehabilitation. Harvest of bone and tissues from distant sites have been associated with limitations and problems, such as donor site morbidity.[30] Therefore, it is crucial to use new sources of cells and tissues to reduce donor site morbidity and challenges faced when harvesting tissue from distant sites. Cells and tissues harvested from maxillary tuberosities previously showed expansion and differentiation potential when used in maxillary sinus augmentation procedures.[31]

Mesenchymal Stem Cells Derived from Gingival Tissues

A subpopulation of MSCs has also been isolated from human gingival tissues (GMSCs), which not only possess stem cell properties but also exhibit potent immunomodulatory and anti-inflammatory effects in tissue.[32,33] GMSCs can be differentiated into adipocytes, osteocytes, chondrocytes, and different lineages of neural cells, such as neuronal and Schwann cells.[33] Most recently, studies have shown that GMSCs can be directly induced into neural progenitor-like cells by using nongenetic approaches. GMSC-derived induced neural progenitor cells show enhanced therapeutic effects on repair/regeneration of injured rat sciatic nerves (see **Fig. 1**).[34] Investigators have also shown that GMSCs are capable of inducing M2 polarization of tissue macrophages.[32] In the presence of GMSCs, macrophages exhibit M2-like macrophage phenotypes characterized by an increased expression of mannose receptors and anti-inflammatory cytokine interleukin 10, while showing decreased expression of proinflammatory cytokine, tumor necrosis factor-α.[32] Additionally, GMSCs are capable of suppressing the activation and function of inflammatory Th-1 and Th-17 cells and promoting the generation of anti-inflammatory regulatory T cells.[32–36] The constellation of effects of GMSCs on both T cells and macrophages results in their application in the therapy for various inflammation-related disease models in rodents, including colitis, contact-allergic dermatitis, oral mucositis, and skin wound healing.[32–36]

CLINICAL TRIALS

Although investigators have attempted to use such cells and technologies to regenerate different tissue types, currently the regenerative modalities using stem cells are not standard therapies approved by major regulatory bodies, such as the Food and Drug Administration. Many such studies are in the stage of animal models or human clinical trials to receive approvals for applications in human subjects.

A review of literature regarding the application of adult MSCs used in maxillary sinus augmentation showed that in the period 2004 to 2011, only 4 randomized controlled trials with numbers of patients ranging from 5 to 26 investigated the efficacy of cell-based methods.[37] A systematic review with meta-analysis of the application of MSCs in maxillary sinus augmentation identified a total of 39 studies (21 human and 18 animal studies) from 2004 to 2014 and demonstrated significant variation in study design, results, and follow-up outcomes.[38] A recent randomized controlled trial (phase 1/phase 2) investigated the total bone and the quality of bone regenerated in maxillary sinus bony defects using autologous cells enriched with CD90$^+$ stem cells and CD14$^+$ monocytes in 30 human participants.[39] In addition to using stem cells to engineer bone, the investigators installed oral implants in the regenerated bone and functionally loaded the implants with prosthetic teeth. Although the radiographic analysis of the regenerated bone did not show a difference in the total bone regenerated between the study and control groups, the bone regenerated using cell-based methods had a higher density. Moreover, the bone core biopsies revealed that stem cell therapy benefited patients with severe defects the most considering the bone volume fraction.[39]

FUTURE PERSPECTIVES

MSCs harvested from oral and craniofacial regions offer easier accessibility with potentially reduced donor site morbidity compared with other grafting sources. These cells have a great potential in differentiation to other cell types and aid in the regeneration of tissues composed of different cell types in the oral and craniofacial region. Before using these cells in human subjects, however, studies need to assess the safety of cell-based therapies, regenerative and differentiation efficacy, and the controlled expansion of these cells in the body. Currently, there are several clinical trials aimed to further study the applications of oral and craniofacial stem cells in regeneration. For instance, the applications of autologous PDLSCs in treating periodontal regeneration and treatment of periodontal disease[40] and the use of SHED cells in the revitalization of immature permanent teeth with necrotic pulp[41] are 2 examples of such trials. Such clinical trials play a pivotal role in shedding light on the potentials of stem cells in tissue engineering and repair of major oral and craniofacial defects with restoring both structure and function.

REFERENCES

1. McGregor IA. The temporalis flap in intra-oral cancer: its role in repairing the post-excisional defect. Br J Plast Surg 1963;16:318–35.
2. Adams GR. The effects of physical attractiveness on the socialization process. In: Lucker GW, Ribbens KA, McNamara JA, editors. Psychological aspects of facial form craniofacial growth. Series Monograph no 11. Ann Arbor (MI): University of Michigan Press; 1981. p. 25–47.
3. Takahashi K, Yamanaka S. Induction of pluripotent stem cells from mouse embryonic and adult fibroblast cultures by defined factors. Cell 2006;126(4):663–76.
4. Alhadlaq A, Mao JJ. Tissue-engineered osteochondral constructs in the shap of an articular condyle. J Bone Joint Surg Am 2005;87:936–44.
5. Guldberg RE, Oest M, Lin AS, et al. Functional integration of tissue-engineered bone constructs. J Musculoskelet Neuronal Interact 2004;4(4):399–400.
6. Akintoye SO, Lam T, Shi S, et al. Skeletal site-specific characterization of orofacial and iliac crest

human bone marrow stromal cells in same individuals. Bone 2006;38(6):758–68.

7. Gronthos S, Brahim J, Li W, et al. Stem cell properties of human dental pulp stem cells. J Dent Res 2002;81(8):531–5.

8. Xu X, Chen C, Akiyama K, et al. Gingivae contain neural-crest- and mesoderm-derived mesenchymal stem cells. J Dent Res 2013;92(9):825–32.

9. Kadakia S, Helman SN, Badhey AK, et al. Treacher Collins syndrome: the genetics of a craniofacial disease. Int J Pediatr Otorhinolaryngol 2014;78(6):893–8.

10. Ricalde P, Magliocca KR, Lee JS. Craniofacial fibrous dysplasia. Oral Maxillofac Surg Clin North Am 2012;24(3):427–41.

11. Ueki Y, Tiziani V, Santanna C, et al. Mutations in the gene encoding c-Abl-binding protein SH3BP2 cause cherubism. Nat Genet 2001;28(2):125–6.

12. Matsubara T, Suardita K, Ishii M, et al. Alveolar bone marrow as a cell source for regenerative medicine: differences between alveolar and iliac bone marrow stromal cells. J Bone Miner Res 2005;20(3):399–409.

13. Chung IH, Yamaza T, Zhao H, et al. Stem cell property of postmigratory cranial neural crest cells and their utility in alveolar bone regeneration and tooth development. Stem Cells 2009;27(4):866–77.

14. Lin Z, Fateh A, Salem DM, et al. Periosteum: biology and applications in craniofacial bone regeneration. J Dent Res 2014;93(2):109–16.

15. Zhao H, Feng J, Ho TV, et al. The suture provides a niche for mesenchymal stem cells of craniofacial bones. Nat Cell Biol 2015;17(4):386–96.

16. Couble ML, Farges JC, Bleicher F, et al. Odontoblast differentiation of human dental pulp cells in explant cultures. Calcif Tissue Int 2000;66(2):129–38.

17. Kuo MY, Lan WH, Lin SK, et al. Collagen gene expression in human dental pulp cell cultures. Arch Oral Biol 1992;37(11):945–52.

18. Tsukamato Y, Fukutani S, Shin-Ike T, et al. Mineralized nodule formation by coltures of human dental pulp-derived fibroblasts. Arch Oral Biol 1992;37(12):1045–55.

19. Shiba H, Nakamura S, Shirakawa M, et al. Effects of basic fibroblast growth factor on proliferation, the expression of osteonectin (SPARC) and alkaline phosphatase, and calcification in cultures of human pulp cells. Dev Biol 1995;170(2):457–66.

20. Gronthos S, Mankani M, Brahim P, et al. Postnatal human dental pulp stem cells (DPSCs) in vitro and in vivo. Proc Natl Acad Sci U S A 2000;97(25):13625–30.

21. Sonoyama W, Liu Y, Fang D, et al. Mesenchymal stem cell-mediated functional tooth regeneration in swine. PLoS One 2006;1:e79–92.

22. Seo BM, Miura M, Gronthos S, et al. Investigation of multipotent postnatal stem cells from human periodontal ligament. Lancet 2004;364(9429):149–55.

23. Liu Y, Zheng Y, Ding G, et al. Periodontal ligament stem cell-mediated treatment for periodontitis in miniature swine. Stem Cells 2008;26(4):1065–73.

24. Ding G, Wang W, Liu Y, et al. Effect of cryopreservation on biological and immunological properties of stem cells from apical papilla. J Cell Physiol 2010;223(2):415–22.

25. Miura M, Gronthos S, Zhao M, et al. SHED: stem cells from human exfoliated deciduous teeth. Proc Natl Acad Sci U S A 2003;100(10):5807–12.

26. Huang GT, Sonoyama W, Liu Y, et al. The hidden treasure in apical papilla: the potential role in pulp/dentin regeneration and bioroot engineering. J Endod 2008;34(6):645–51.

27. Sakai VT, Zhang Z, Dong Z, et al. SHED differentiate into functional odontoblasts and endothelium. J Dent Res 2010;89(8):791–6.

28. Zheng Y, Liu Y, Zhang CM, et al. Stem cells from deciduous tooth repair mandibular defect in swine. J Dent Res 2009;88(3):249–54.

29. Xu J, Zheng Z, Fang D, et al. Mesenchymal stromal cell-based treatment of jaw osteoradionecrosis in swine. Cell Transplant 2012;21(8):1679–86.

30. Zouhary KJ. Bone graft harvesting from distant sites: concepts and techniques. Oral Maxillofac Surg Clin North Am 2010;22(3):301–16.

31. Springer IN, Nocini PF, Schlegel KA, et al. Two techniques for the preparation of cell-scaffold constructs suitable for sinus augmentation: steps into clinical application. Tissue Eng 2006;12:2649–56.

32. Zhang Q-Z, Su W-R, Shi S-H, et al. Human gingiva-derived mesenchymal stem cells elicit polarization of M2 macrophages and enhance cutaneous wound Healing. Stem Cells 2010;28(10):1856–68.

33. Zhang Q, Shi S, Liu Y, et al. Mesenchymal stem cells derived from human gingiva are capable of immunomodulatory functions and ameliorate inflammation-related tissue destruction in experimental colitis. J Immunol 2009;183(12):7787–98.

34. Zhang Q, Nguyen P, Xu Q, et al. Neural progenitor-like cells induced from human gingiva-derived mesenchymal stem cells regulate myelination of schwann cells in rat sciatic nerve regeneration. Stem Cells Transl Med 2016. [pii:sctm.2016-0177]; [Epub ahead of print].

35. Su WR, Zhang QZ, Shi SH, et al. Human gingiva-derived mesenchymal stromal cells attenuate contact hypersensitivity via prostaglandin E2-dependent mechanisms. Stem Cells 2011;29(11):1849–60.

36. Zhang QZ, Nguyen AL, Yu WH, et al. Human oral mucosa and gingiva: a unique reservoir for mesenchymal stem cells. J Dent Res 2012;91(11):1011–8.

37. Mangano FG, Tettamanti L, Sammons RL, et al. Maxillary sinus augmentation with adult mesenchymal stem cells: a review of the current literature. Oral Surg Oral Med Oral Pathol Oral Radiol 2013;115(6):717–23.

38. Mangano FG, Colombo M, Caprioglio A. Mesenchymal stem cells in maxillary sinus augmentation: a systematic review with meta-analysis. World J Stem Cells 2015;7(6):976–91.

39. Kaigler D, Avila-Ortiz G, Travan S, et al. Bone engineering of maxillary sinus bone deficiencies using enriched CD90þ stem cell therapy: a randomized clinical trial. J Bone Miner Res 2015;30:1206–16.

40. Wang S. Periodontal regeneration of chronic periodontal disease patients receiving stem cells injection therapy. Bethesda (MD): National Library of Medicine (US); 2015. Available at: https://clinicaltrials.gov/ct2/show/NCT02523651?term=dpsc&rank=1.

41. Yan J, Fourth Military Medical University. Revitalization of immature permanent teeth with necrotic pulps using SHED cells. Bethesda (MD): National Library of Medicine (US); 2013. Available at: https://clinicaltrials.gov/ct2/show/NCT01814436?term=shed+cells&rank=1.

42. Kerkis I, Ambrosio CE, Kerkis A, et al. Early transplantation of human immature dental pulp stem cells from baby teeth to golden retriever muscular dystrophy (GRMD) dogs: local or systemic? J Transl Med 2008;6:35. http://dx.doi.org/10.1186/1479-5876-6-35.

43. Gandia C, Armiñan A, García-Verdugo JM, et al. Human dental pulp stem cells improve left ventricular function, induce angiogenesis, and reduce infarct size in rats with acute myocardial infarction. Stem Cells 2008;26:638–45.

44. Monteiro BG, Serafim RC, Melo GB, et al. Human immature dental pulp stem cells share key characteristic features with limbal stem cells. Cell Prolif 2009;42:587–94.

45. Gomes JA, Geraldes Monteiro B, Melo GB, et al. Corneal reconstruction with tissue-engineered cell sheets composed of human immature dental pulp stem cells. Invest Ophthalmol Vis Sci 2010;51:1408–14.

46. Wang J, Wang X, Sun Z, et al. Stem cells from human-exfoliated deciduous teeth can differentiate into dopaminergic neuron-like cells. Stem Cells Dev 2010;19:1375–83.

47. Wang F, Yu M, Yan X, et al. Gingiva-derived mesenchymal stem cell-mediated therapeutic approach for bone tissue regeneration. Stem Cells Dev 2011;20:2093–102.

48. Zhang J, Jiao K, Zhang M, et al. Occlusal effects on longitudinal bone alterations of the temporomandibular joint. J Dent Res 2013;92:253–9.

Tissue Engineering for Vertical Ridge Reconstruction

Neel Patel, DMD, MD[a], Beomjune Kim, DMD, MD[b],
Waleed Zaid, DDS, FRCD(c), MSc[b],
Daniel Spagnoli, DDS, MS, PhD[c],*

KEYWORDS

- Vertical alveolar ridge augmentation • Vertical ridge reconstruction
- Tissue engineering for vertical ridge defects • Bone grafting for vertical ridge augmentation
- Bioactive agents for vertical defect reconstruction

KEY POINTS

- Tissue engineering represents an important advancement in vertical ridge augmentation and has the potential to increase success rates significantly.
- Regenerative medicine techniques are used in conjunction with traditional vertical reconstructive procedures to enhance postoperative results and improve outcomes.
- Research continues to provide better and more reliable bioactive materials, which serve to advance the future of reconstructive maxillofacial surgery.

INTRODUCTION

It is a well-known fact that regaining vertical dimension in dentoalveolar reconstructive surgery is a difficult task. Many techniques have been outlined in the literature over the years. However, these have been plagued by issues, such as resorption and relapse, which are usually caused by such problems as soft tissue shrinkage and lack of basal bone stock to support the grafting material. The advent of dental implants and the concept of osseointegration, and improved techniques in implant dentistry, have improved outcomes in oral rehabilitation involving vertical bone defects. Evolving research on newer and more reliable biomaterials, including the use of bioactive factors, such as bone morphogenic proteins (BMPs), have contributed to a significant advancement in alveolar ridge augmentation.

Traditionally, multiple surgical techniques are outlined that have been used to achieve an increase in vertical bone height. Autogenous grafts are currently the gold standard, given that they are the only material that has true osteogenic potential in addition to its osteoinductive and osteoconductive capabilities.[1–3] However, autologous bone grafting does present with several inherent disadvantages including donor site morbidities (second site of pain, swelling, and other site-specific complications), increased surgical time (increasing rates of infection), and lengthier hospital stays.[4] Each of the current methods of vertical

Disclosure Statement: The authors have nothing to disclose.
[a] Department of Oral and Maxillofacial Surgery, Louisiana State University Health Sciences Center, 1100 Florida Ave, Box 220, Room 5303, New Orleans, LA 70119, USA; [b] Department of Oral and Maxillofacial Surgery, Louisiana State University Health Sciences Center, 1100 Florida Avenue, Box 220, Room 5303, New Orleans, LA, USA; [c] Private Practice, Brunswick Oral and Maxillofacial Surgery, 621-B North Fodale Avenue, Southport, NC 28461, USA
* Corresponding author.
E-mail address: omfs.spagnoli@gmail.com

ridge augmentation has found its unique niche in reconstructive maxillofacial surgery and each presents with its own indications and limitations with regards to how much bone height is gained. Examples of current methods include corticocancellous block grafts, distraction osteogenesis, and the tent pole technique, among various others. Reconstruction of the largest defects has been fairly successful using distraction osteogenesis, but even this technique requires a sufficient width and height of native bone to ensure a sufficient bone mass to translate.[5] The authors present several cases where tissue engineering principles were combined with traditional vertical ridge augmentation techniques to achieve improved clinical outcomes.

CASE PRESENTATIONS
Case 1

A 58-year-old woman with an unremarkable past medical history presented with ill-fitting dentures. The patient wanted to explore the option of implant-retained prosthetic rehabilitation as a more desirable permanent long-term solution. On performing a thorough work-up including clinical photographs, orthopantomogram, and lateral cephalometric analysis we see that the patient presented with significant maxillary pseudodeficiency secondary to severe vertical and horizontal resorption of the alveolar ridge (**Figs. 1–3**) that was compensated for by the thickness of the maxillary denture flange (**Fig. 4**). This case is not amenable to standard vertical augmentation because this would not correct the interarch relationship and thus would not result in a desirable esthetic and functional outcome.[6] The decision was made to use Le Fort I osteotomy and downgraft with advancement to correct the horizontal and vertical components of the atrophic maxilla in this patient, and the unfavorable interarch relationship (**Figs. 5 and 6**). A combination of recombinant human BMP (rhBMP)-2, iliac crest cancellous autograft, and freeze-dried bone allograft (FDBA) was used as the grafting construct (**Figs. 7–12**). At 4 months postoperatively, a significant increase in vertical height is seen. The patient was deemed ready for the second stage of treatment at 6 months postoperatively, and a Simplant-guided (Dentsply, Mölndal, Sweden) implant surgery was performed to place eight maxillary endosseous implants (**Figs. 13–18**). Primary stability was achieved in all of the implants, with no failures. An excellent anterior esthetic result is seen at the patient's prosthetic try-in appointment (**Fig. 19**).

Disadvantages of this technique include an increased cost of procedure, an extended hospital

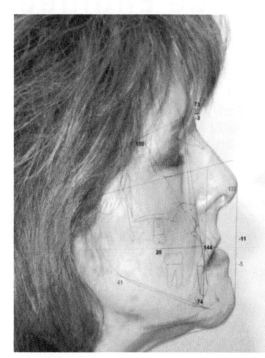

Fig. 1. Patient seen with evident maxillomandibular dysharmony.

stay, and the inherent morbidity of the procedure itself. These are factors that need to be considered and discussed with the patient. Complications, such as palatal fracture (2%) and postoperative sinusitis (3%), have been reported, and the rarer issues of massive hemorrhage and blindness.[7] It has been advocated that these be done in a two-stage process, with implant placement done at a later stage because of unpredictable bone resorption and plate removal at time of implant placement.[8]

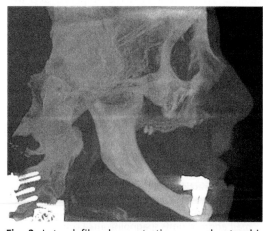

Fig. 2. Lateral film demonstrating severely atrophic maxilla.

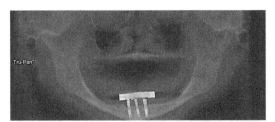

Fig. 3. Orthopantomogram showing loss of vertical height of maxilla.

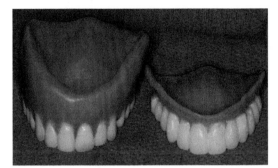

Fig. 4. Thick denture flanges to compensate for severe maxillary deficiency.

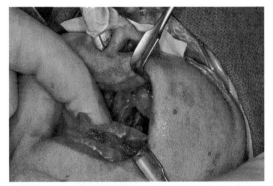

Fig. 5. Le Fort I downfracture.

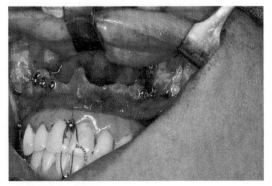

Fig. 6. Rigid fixation.

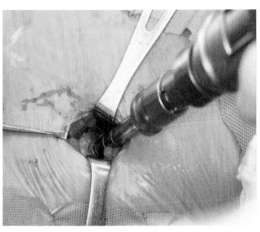

Fig. 7. Trephine to harvest anterior iliac bone graft.

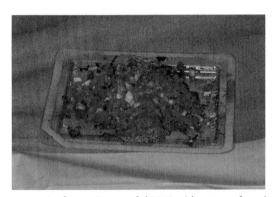

Fig. 8. Grafting mixture of rhBMP with autograft and FDBA.

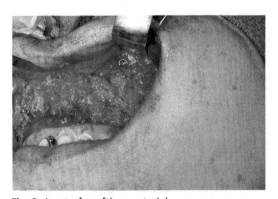

Fig. 9. Inset of grafting material.

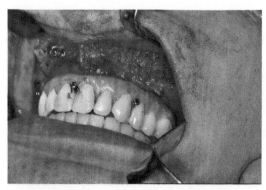

Fig. 10. Fixation of complete upper denture to maxilla.

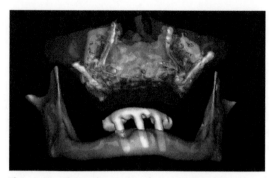

Fig. 13. Three-dimensional representation of reconstruction.

Case 2

A 47-year-old man presented to the clinic desiring dental rehabilitation with implants after losing teeth #12, 13, and 14. The patient requested individual restorations with three maxillary implants. As seen in the initial orthopantomogram (**Fig. 20**), the patient presented with a significant deficiency in vertical bone height, only having 3 mm of native bone in the most deficient areas. The treatment plan was to perform a sinus lift, complete a bone graft using tissue engineering, and simultaneously place dental implants. The sinus lift was performed using the lateral window approach (**Fig. 21**) and the schneiderian membrane was carefully elevated to make room for the grafting material. The next step was the placement of three endosseous dental implants to replace teeth #12, 13, and 14 (**Fig. 22**). We then proceeded to use a combination of rhBMP and demineralized FDBA to augment the maxillary sinus, packing around the implants (**Fig. 23**). The postoperative orthopantomogram shows successful placement of the implants with the grafted maxillary sinus (**Fig. 24**). The patient received his final restorations 6 months later (**Fig. 25**). This case demonstrates successful use of tissue engineering techniques simultaneously with implant placement.

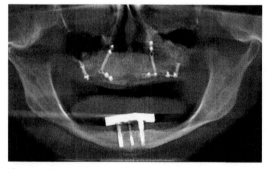

Fig. 11. Postoperative orthopantomogram showing significant increase in bone height.

Case 3

An 18-year-old boy presented with a large mandibular ameloblastoma extending from the right parasymphysis to the left posterior body region (**Fig. 26**). Segmental mandibulectomy with 1 cm normal bony margins was planned based on the pathology. After thorough discussion of multiple reconstructive options, the decision was to use a vascularized free fibula flap. Traditionally, the fibula is placed at the level of the inferior border of the mandible. However, the fibula is generally less than 15 mm thick, introducing a significant height discrepancy with the native mandible,

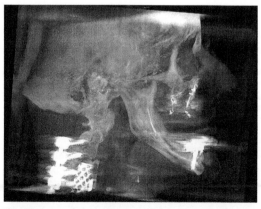

Fig. 12. Lateral cephalogram showing improved maxillomandibular relationship.

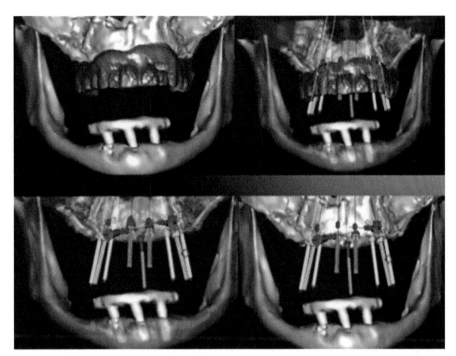

Fig. 14. Simplant-guided implant surgery planning.

particularly in the anterior region. This theoretically increases the cantilever effect on the prospective prosthesis, leading to potential early dental implant failure. Several solutions have been developed to overcome the vertical discrepancy from fibula free flap reconstruction including distraction osteogenesis of the fibula segment, the double-barrel fibula, and higher fibula positioning in the defect.

Satisfactory outcomes from distraction osteogenesis and double-barrel fibula have been reported in the literature but their shortcomings include the need for multiple surgeries, issues with patient compliance, and the inability to reconstruct a long-span mandibular defect. The authors decided to place the fibula at the level of the alveolus for our patient, which provides an ideal maxillomandibular relationship and a platform for immediate implant placement (**Fig. 27**). The inferior defect was filled with a tissue-engineered graft composed of rhBMP-2, anterior iliac crest autograft, and bone marrow aspirate concentrate (BMAC) for restoration of the facial contour (**Fig. 28**). Immediate postoperative computed tomography showed a satisfactory maxillomandibular relationship and facial contour

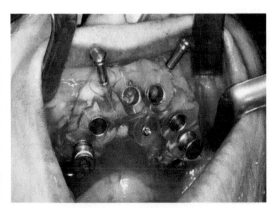

Fig. 15. Use of Simplant guide Intraoperatively.

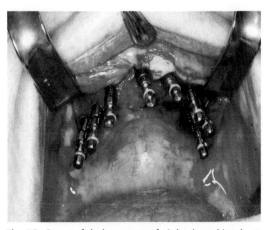

Fig. 16. Successful placement of eight dental implants using Simplant-guided technique.

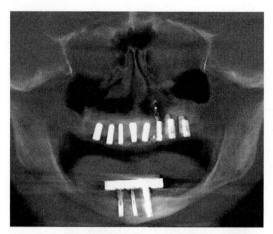

Fig. 17. Postoperative orthopantomogram showing excellent positioning of implants within grafted maxilla.

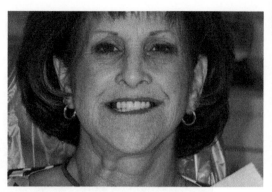

Fig. 19. Patient at prosthetic try-in visit, showing excellent esthetic result.

(Fig. 29). Dental implant placement and vestibulo-plasty were performed at 6 months (Fig. 30). An orthopantomogram taken at 12 months showed complete consolidation of the fibula bone and tissue engineered graft and impressive remodeling into the native mandibular shape (Fig. 31). A traditional crown and bridge type prosthesis was delivered without any cantilevering effect (Fig. 32). The patient has been followed for more than 2 years without any implant or prosthesis failure.

Case 4

A 57-year-old woman with a history of facial trauma presented with missing maxillary anterior teeth from #6 to #11 and a severely resorbed pre-maxillary ridge (Fig. 33). The patient desired fixed crowns and bridges and thus ridge augmentation

with four implants was initially planned. Virtual surgical planning was performed to simulate a prospective prosthesis and to estimate the vertical and horizontal deficiency (Fig. 34). A patient-specific mesh was prefabricated on the stereographic model as a scaffold for the grafting procedure (Fig. 35). The surgery proceeded with exposure of the maxillary defect (Fig. 36). Several small burr holes were created through the maxillary buccal cortex to facilitate neovascularization of the graft. The mesh was then placed to cover the defect. Subsequently, BMAC was obtained from the iliac crest using the BMAC system (HarvestTech, Lakewood, CO) with the specially designed trocars and aspiration needles. BMA was centrifuged to isolate the mesenchymal stem cells (MSC; 1.1 million cells/mL can be obtained). BMA was mixed with Infuse (rhBMP-2, Medtronic, Minneapolis, MN), and particulate mineralized allograft from the University of Miami Tissue Bank (Miami, FL) (see Fig. 6). This mixture was placed into the defect under the mesh, which was then secured with two screws on the buccal side (Fig. 37). The incision was then closed with interrupted 4–0 chromic gut sutures in a tension-free manner (Fig. 38).

The patient was brought back 5 months later for implant placement. The patient changed her mind and decided to pursue individual implants for the missing six teeth. The Simplant software (Dentsply) was used for virtual placement of dental implants and a surgical guide was provided (Fig. 39). A crestal incision was made to expose the new alveolar ridge. The mesh was completely incorporated into the bone. Only a small portion of the mesh at the crest had to be removed to place the dental implants. The surgical guide was placed on the remaining maxillary teeth as a reference. Dental implants were placed following the manufacturer's drilling sequence with adequate

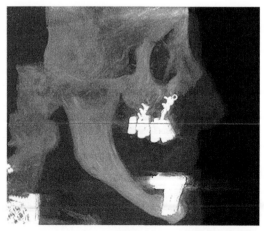

Fig. 18. Lateral cephalogram showing implant placement.

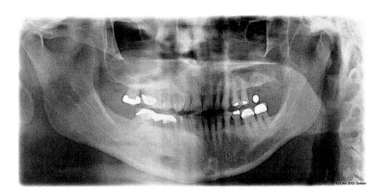

Fig. 20. Pneumatized left maxillary sinus.

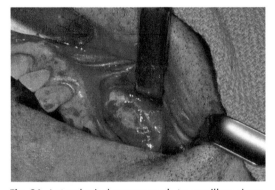

Fig. 21. Lateral window approach to maxillary sinus.

torque values (**Fig. 40**). Healing abutments were placed in the new bone and primary stability of the implants was obtained. The patient received crowns 6 weeks postimplant surgery to her esthetic and functional satisfaction (**Fig. 41**).

Case 5

A 44-year-old man with previously placed left maxillary subperiosteal implant (**Fig. 42**) presents with pain, infection, and purulent discharge in the area of the implant. Initial treatment was removal of the subperiosteal implant and debridement. This resulted in a large defect in the left maxillary alveolar ridge (**Fig. 43**), which did not allow for new implant placement. Using the concept of tissue engineering, delayed reconstruction was performed using rhBMP and FDBA, which served as the scaffold for cellular ingrowth and for the ideal contour of the future construct (**Fig. 44**). In this case one can see that excellent restoration

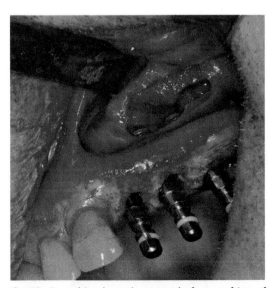

Fig. 22. Dental implant placement before grafting of maxillary sinus.

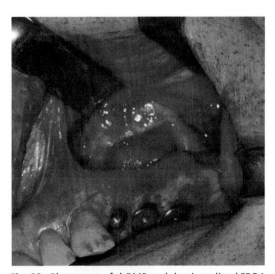

Fig. 23. Placement of rhBMP and demineralized FDBA in maxillary sinus around implants.

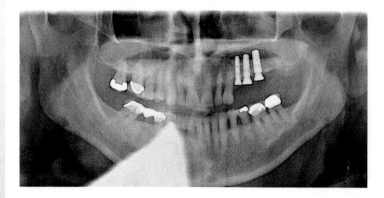

Fig. 24. Postoperative orthopanto-mogram with implants in excellent position.

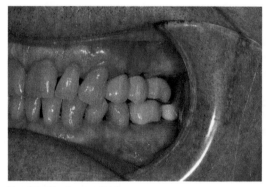

Fig. 25. Final restoration.

of vertical ridge height was obtained using this technique (**Fig. 45**), with subsequent implant placement (**Fig. 46**) and final restoration (**Fig. 47**). Subperiosteal implants were initially introduced in the 1940s; however, now they are rarely used because of their unreliable success rate, along with increased predictability of modern bone grafting techniques, and the availability of alternative options, such as zygomatic implants. The original concept behind using these implants was to increase the retention and stability of complete dentures.

Case 6

A 64-year-old woman presented for dental implant rehabilitation of the left mandibular ridge. The patient had been missing teeth #18, 19, and 20 for

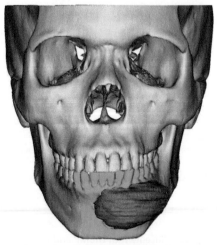
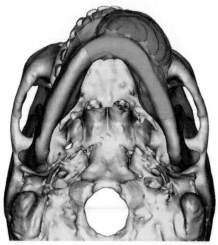

Fig. 26. Three-dimensional views of mandibular ameloblastoma.

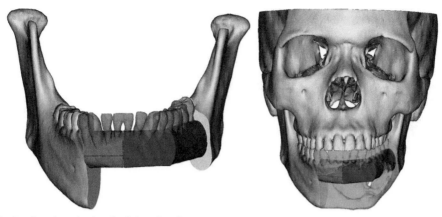

Fig. 27. Fibula placed at the level of the alveolus.

many years and was left with a vertically deficient left mandibular alveolar ridge (**Fig. 48**). The patient initially presented with 6 mm of bone available for implant placement. The decision was to perform vertical augmentation using tissue engineering technique simultaneously with implant placement. A guided implant surgery was performed (**Fig. 49**) with supracrestal implant placement (**Fig. 50**), in preparation for bony augmentation. A resorbable membrane was used in this case and was initially tacked down on the lingual surface (**Fig. 51**). RhBMP was used and was wrapped around the implants (**Fig. 52**); allogenic cancellous bone was placed superiorly (**Fig. 53**), with the mesh then secured with screws onto the buccal surface (**Fig. 54**). The tissues were well released and a passive closure was achieved (**Fig. 55**). Postoperative imaging reveals adequate implant placement with bone grafting to the appropriate height and width (**Fig. 56**). Photographs at 4 months postoperatively showed excellent healing of the soft tissues (**Fig. 57**). At 6 months, the site was reentered for the second stage, showing incorporation of the membrane and good bony height covering the implants (**Fig. 58**). Good osseointegration was confirmed (**Fig. 59**) and healing caps were placed (**Fig. 60**). The final photograph shows excellent restoration in place (**Fig. 61**).

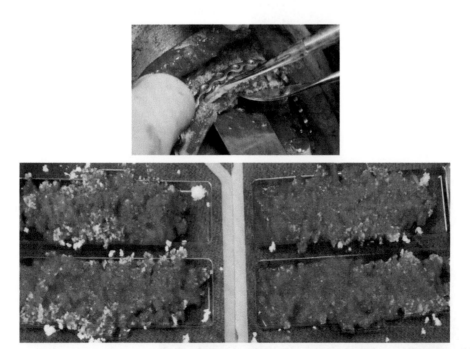

Fig. 28. Tissue engineered graft composed of morselized anterior iliac crest bone, BMAC, and rhBMP-2. This graft was packed into the inferior mandibular defect below the fibula segment.

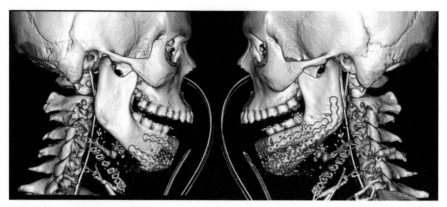

Fig. 29. Segmental mandibular reconstruction completed with superior fibula segment and inferior tissue-engineered bone graft on immediate postoperative computed tomography.

DISCUSSION
Basic Principles of Tissue Engineering

There have been significant advancements in techniques of tissue engineering, with a wide use throughout the fields of medicine, dentistry, and surgery. The goal of tissue engineering is to regenerate damaged, and sometimes missing tissues by combining cells from the body with highly porous scaffold biomaterials that act as templates for tissue regeneration and guide the growth of new tissue.[9] These biologic substitutes that are produced ultimately restore and maintain function.[10] The so-called "tissue engineering triangle" (**Fig. 62**) dictates that three major components need to be present for successful tissue regeneration: (1) a source of cells, (2) signaling molecules, and (3) a matrix.[11] This forms the basic construct from which de novo tissues are regenerated for reconstruction and repair of multiple defects and deformities. In regards to bone, there are materials that are osteoinductive (ability of a grafting material to induce stem cells to differentiate into mature bone cells), osteoconductive (a physical property

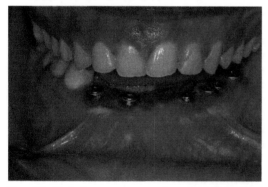

Fig. 30. Clinical appearance after dental implant placement and vestibuloplasty at 6 months.

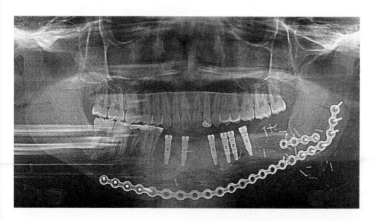

Fig. 31. Orthopantomogram taken at 12 months. Dental implants were placed in the interim period.

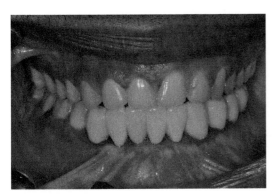

Fig. 32. Final prosthesis.

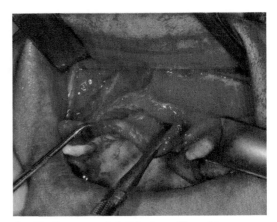

Fig. 36. Exposure of deficient maxillary ridge.

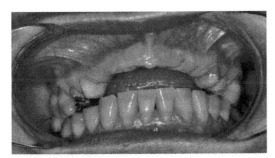

Fig. 33. Anterior maxillary defect.

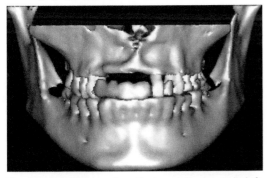

Fig. 34. Estimation of vertical and horizontal deficiency with three-dimensional imaging.

of the graft to serve as a scaffold or matrix for viable bone healing), and osteogenic (ability of the grating material to itself produce new bone),[12] as seen in **Table 1**.

Bioactive Agents

The use of bioactive products, such as rhBMP, has significantly increased the success rate of bone regeneration.[13,14] BMP-2 in particular has shown to have the highest osteinductive properties and is thus important in the proliferation and differentiation of mesenchymal progenitor cells into osteoblasts.[15,16] BMPs are part of the transforming growth factor-β superfamily that was first investigated by Urist[17] and were later isolated and shown to induce endochondral and intramembraneous bone formation from MSC.[18,19] The main issue with the use of rhBMP has been the lack of a suitable delivery system, or scaffold, which should be osteoconductive, safe, biocompatible, have the appropriate three-dimensional support and structure, and should not adversely affect the regenerative capabilities of the grafting material.[20,21] The most commonly used carrier is the absorbable collagen sponge (ACS), derived from highly purified bovine tendon type-I collagen, which has been shown to provide a good scaffold for delivery

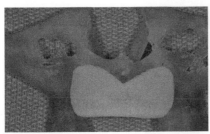
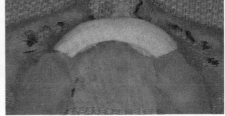

Fig. 35. A prefabricated mesh.

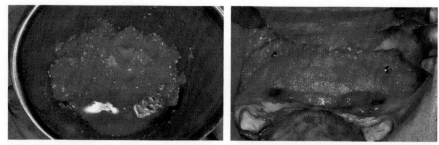

Fig. 37. Mixture of BMAC, allograft, and rhBMP-2, and placement of tissue-engineered graft under the mesh.

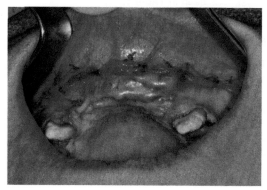

Fig. 38. Tension-free closure.

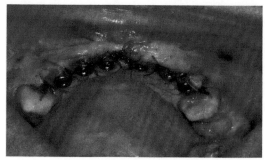

Fig. 40. Implants placed at proper vertical position for crown-and-bridge type prosthesis.

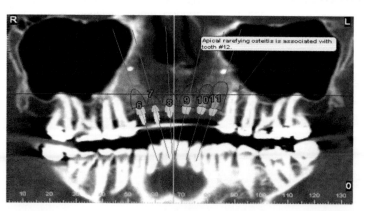

Fig. 39. Virtual planning of implant placement. The vertical height gain is appreciated on the image.

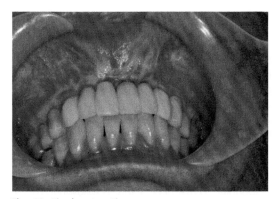

Fig. 41. Final restoration.

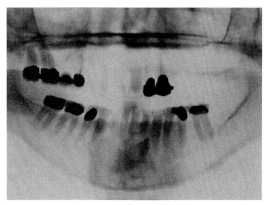

Fig. 43. Severe left maxillary resorption after subperiosteal implant removal and debridement.

of rhBMP in the setting of bony ridge defects. The main disadvantage is the lack of structural stability because it is often compressed by the overlying soft tissues.[22] Nonetheless, the rhBMP/ACS construct has yielded successful results and has been used widely in reconstructive maxillofacial surgery.

A randomized clinical trial studied the use of this construct in combination with crushed cancellous freeze-dried allogenic bone and platelet-rich plasma, and compared it with the use of 100% autogenous bone graft in large vertical defects of the maxillary alveolar ridge. The results of the study concluded that the use of this so-called "composite graft" yielded equal results to autogenous bone grafting in regards to bone regeneration. In addition, the rhBMP/ACS construct has been used in maxillary sinus augmentation procedures, and has been met with significant success. De novo bone that was formed with this construct contained a vascular marrow space;

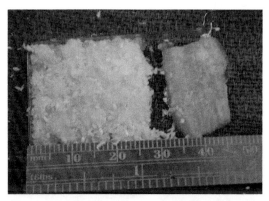

Fig. 44. Use of BMP with FDBA (250–800 μm).

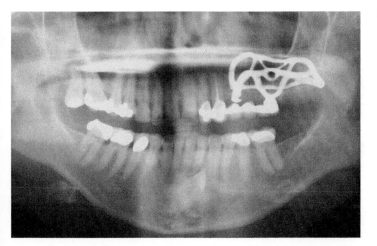

Fig. 42. Subperiosteal implant.

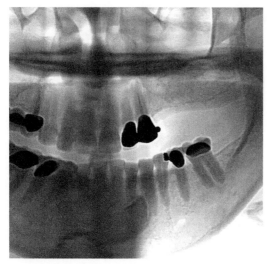

Fig. 45. Postoperative orthopantomogram 6 months after bone grafting, showing excellent restoration of bone height.

had a moderate degree of new trabecular bone containing both woven (initial) bone and lamellar (mature) bone; had a higher proportion of osteoblasts than osteoclasts, consistent with overall bone growth; showed little to no histologic evidence of inflammation; and no collagen matrix was detected at 6 months to 1 year postoperatively (**Fig. 63**). In another prospective study, the rhBMP/ACS construct was shown to increase bone levels by almost 8 mm within the maxillary sinus, and was also denser bone than the bone graft group, suggesting that the bone formed was also responding to mechanical forces following Wolff's law, which states that bone that is subjected to a load remodels to become thicker and stronger, whereas if load decreases, bone becomes less dense and weaker as a result of a lack of stimulus for remodeling.[23,24] One of the well-known drawbacks with rhBMP was the significant facial edema that was induced postoperatively, caused by the

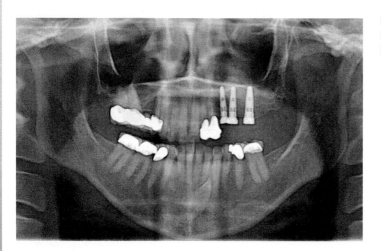

Fig. 46. Postoperative orthopantomogram immediately after implant placement.

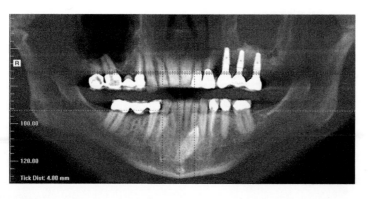

Fig. 47. Cone beam computed tomography 5 years postoperative showing final restorations, with maintained bone height, consolidation of the bone graft, and excellent radiographic osseointegration of the dental implants.

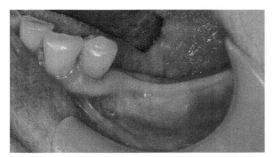

Fig. 48. Deficient left mandibular alveolar ridge.

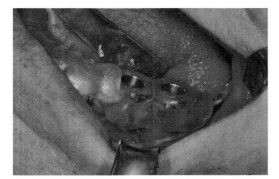

Fig. 49. Implant guide in place.

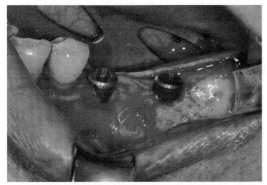

Fig. 50. Implant placement at appropriate height relative to adjacent teeth.

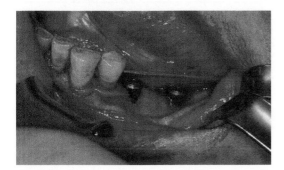

Fig. 51. Resorbable mesh secured onto lingual surface before placement of bone graft material.

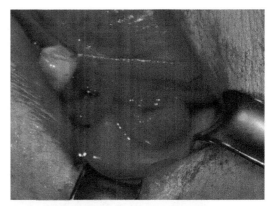

Fig. 52. rhBMP placed around implants.

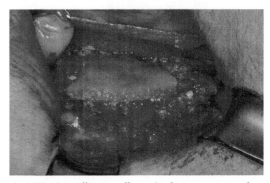

Fig. 53. Cancelleous allogenic bone to complete augmentation of ridge.

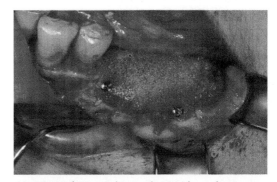

Fig. 54. Graft secured into place with mesh.

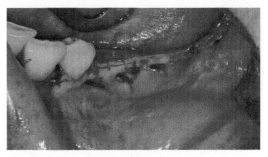

Fig. 55. Passive closure achieved.

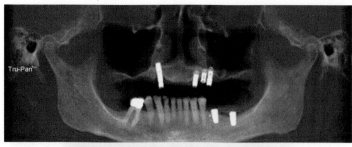

Fig. 56. Immediate postoperative imaging showing adequate bone augmentation.

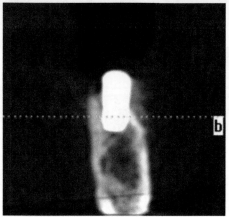

influx of fluid and cells from chemotaxis and neo-vascularization during the healing process.[25]

Another delivery system for rhBMP that has been studied is the use of a resorbable bioactive ceramic (SCPC50). One of the noted advantages over previously used carriers is that it is able to regulate the long-term release kinetics of the rhBMP, allowing it to be released at a slow rate, accelerating the synchronized bone formation and resorption of graft material.[26] In addition, the vascularity of bone and its maturation are enhanced by the silicon, calcium, and phosphorus contents of the ceramic.[27,28] Studies have shown that this construct was capable of achieving a 6-mm-plus gain in vertical bone height and 93.50% defect fill over a period of 8 weeks.[26]

MESENCHYMAL STEM CELLS

The use of pluripotent MSCs in the bone marrow stroma has been well established in the orthopedic and neurosurgical literature in relation to use in spinal fusion.[29] In recent years it has also been studied in oral and maxillofacial surgery most often

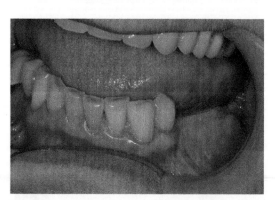

Fig. 57. Four months postoperatively showing good healing.

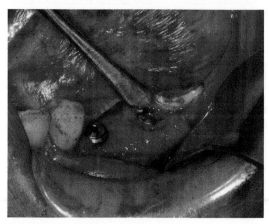

Fig. 58. Second-stage surgery at 6 months showing good bony restoration around implants.

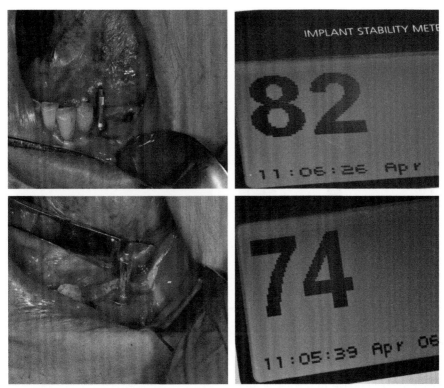

Fig. 59. Implant stability quotient values showing good osseotintegration of implants.

in sinus augmentation procedures. The MSCs are harvested using a bone marrow biopsy needle (**Fig. 64**) from the pelvic bone about 2 cm inferolateral to the posterior superior iliac spine.[30] The BMAC system is used, and it can be done in the operating room.[31] Similar to rhBMP, these MSCs require a suitable delivery system in the form of an osteoconductive scaffold. A suitable construct had been made by using beta-tri-calcium-phosphate (b-TCP) in combination with

hydroxyapatite, which had been shown to induce bone formation in large defects in long bones.[32,33] This same construct has been used in sinus augmentation grafting procedures before implant placement, and yielded clinically successful results.[34] The use of platelet-rich plasma in combination with b-TCP and MSCs, as the source of osteoinductive growth factors, has also been studied in regards to maxillary sinus augmentation and onlay grafting for vertical augmentation, with

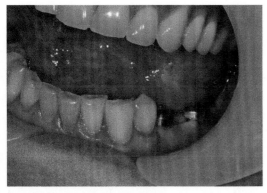

Fig. 60. Second stage completed.

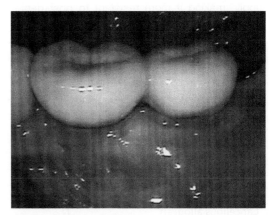

Fig. 61. Final restoration.

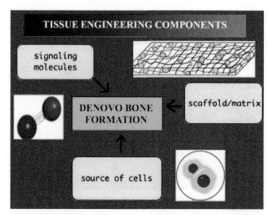

Fig. 62. Tissue engineering basics.

simultaneous implant placement.[35] In fact, this was engineered into an injectable form of grafting material, which enhances its ease of use intraoperatively.

MODIFIED TENT POLE TECHNIQUE

The atrophic mandible presents its own unique set of challenges in reconstructive maxillofacial surgery. A mandibular vertical height of less than 2 cm (20 mm) is universally considered atrophic, and presents with characteristic anatomic and physiologic features, such as hypovascularity, which might contribute to tooth and alveolar process loss. The atrophic resorption patterns also contribute to the consistent anatomic changes, such as prominent mylohyoid and internal oblique ridges, which are covered with a thin mucosal lining, contributing to an increased risk of soft tissue breakdown and dehiscence. These anatomic changes happen secondary to a deficiency in blood supply from the lack of muscle attachments in those areas, whereas the areas that have a healthy musculature show an increased blood supply, making it more resistant to post–dental

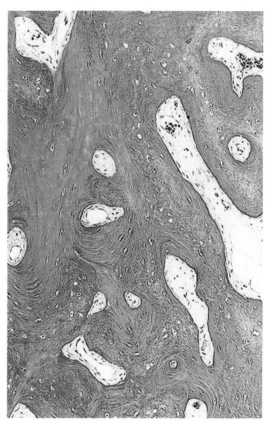

Fig. 63. Hematoxylin-eosin stain 32 weeks postoperatively, demonstrating de novo bone from rhBMP/ACS construct. Original magnification ×10.

extraction resorption.[36] An important concept that reconstructive surgeons need to understand is that atrophic mandibles depend heavily on periosteal blood supply because of the narrowing of the inferior alveolar artery.[37,38]

Cawood and his group from the United Kingdom found that alveolar bone resorption seemed to have a predictable pattern: class I, dentate; class II, immediately postextraction;

Table 1
Properties of different bone grafting materials

	Osteogenic	Osteoinductive	Osteoconductive
Cancellous autograft	Y	Y	Y
Bone marrow aspirate	Y	Y	N
Demineralized bone matrix	N	Y	Y
Bone morphogenic proteins	N	Y	Depends on carrier
Platelet-rich plasma	N	Y	N
Ceramics	N	N	Y
Cancellous allograft	N	N	Y

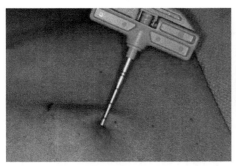
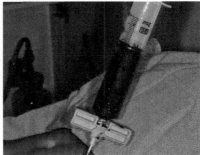

Fig. 64. Harvesting of MSCs using BMAC system from iliac crest.

class III, well-rounded ridge form, adequate in height and width; class IV, knife-edge ridge form, adequate in height and inadequate in width; class V, flat ridge form, inadequate in height and width; and class VI, depressed ridge form, with some basilar bone loss evident.[39] This classification has more relevance to implant dentistry because it gives the operator an idea of whether an adjunctive bone graft would be necessary (class IV and V). Marx and colleagues[40] published a novel soft tissue matrix expansion also known as the "tent pole," where the dental implants effectively "tent" the soft tissue envelope up to

maintain the bone graft volume and prevent soft tissue collapse (**Fig. 65**). The original description used an extraoral submental approach and the bone graft material of choice was the anterior iliac crest bone graft, with four to five implants placed (each one 15 mm in height), with a 1-cm interimplant distance. Primary stability was obtained by engaging the inferior border of the mandible with the implants. Autogenous corticocancellous bone graft is then packed around the implants. The authors have found that the addition of rhBMP in the tent pole technique had a favorable impact on bone healing and allowed substitution

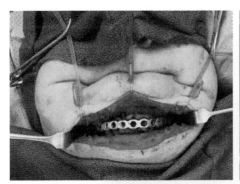
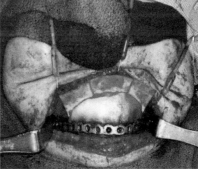
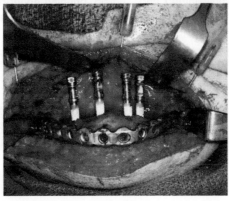

Fig. 65. Classic tent pole technique with addition of rhBMP.

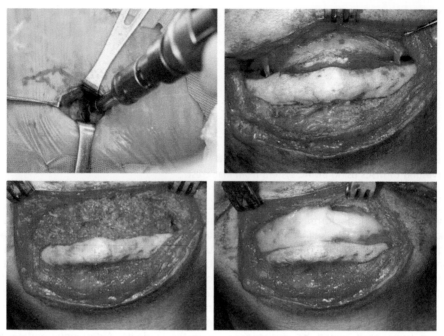

Fig. 66. Modified tent pole: using trephine and rhBMP with rib graft serving as lingual strut.

of the posterior iliac crest as a donor site with the anterior iliac crest bone graft because of the enhanced osteoinduction that happens with rhBMP. Furthermore, the authors rarely use the classical anterior iliac crest bone grafting approach, instead opting for the trephine to harvest bone from the anterior iliac crest (**Fig. 66**), with excellent increase in vertical bone height and final implant placement (**Fig. 67**). In our patient population, this translated to less donor site morbidity and earlier mobilization.

Many surgeons have modified Marx's original tent pole technique, and some have replaced dental implants with bone screws; this modification seemed to improve the buccolingual orientation of the final implant placement, because the dental implants would be placed at a second procedure, when all of the bone has consolidated, and the position of the implants is more ideal. A second advantage of this modification is that it allows the use of surgical implant guides, especially if a maxillary prosthesis exists. Another commonly used method is the use of a titanium mesh to tent the soft tissue and maintain the bone graft and the contour of the ridge. However, the main disadvantage of this technique is that the surgical site must be re-entered to remove the titanium mesh before implant placement. This has presented its own set of challenges, especially when the graft grows over the mesh, and the procedure requires excessive soft tissue reflection.

OTHER AVAILABLE MATERIALS AND TECHNIQUES

Research is constantly advancing the health care field, bringing about novel techniques and materials into patient care. Another bioactive agent

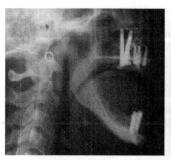
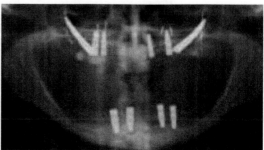

Fig. 67. Increase of 10 mm in bone height, with placement of four mandibular implants, each 13 mm in length.

that has been studied in maxillofacial reconstructive surgery is recombinant human platelet-derived growth factor. This is a product of platelets and functions as a chemotactic and mitogenic factor for osteoblasts, and is critical for angiogenesis, and thus can be applied to treating ridge defects.[41] This growth factor has been combined with several different types of grafting materials and carriers, such as mineralized and demineralized FDBA,[42] xenograft (specifically deproteinized bovine block graft), equine block graft,[43–45] and bTCP,[46] in multiple case series and has been shown to help produce intact woven and lamellar bone contributing to an increase in vertical ridge height in humans, which was of appropriate quality to accommodate the placement of dental implants at a second stage.

The concept of engineered heterotopic bone formation has also been studied; however, this has not yet gained much notoriety. In 2004 it was studied in the reconstruction of large segmental mandibular defects by way of an engineered growth of a mandibular transplant within a muscular environment (in this case the latissimus dorsi muscle) with the help of BMPs, with subsequent free tissue transfer of the bone-muscle flap approximately 7 weeks later.[47] A prefabricated titanium mesh was filled with bone mineral blocks, BMPs, and the patient's own bone marrow. Although a clinically successful result was obtained, this procedure may not be as cost effective as some of the more traditional and established methods of free tissue transfer for mandibular reconstruction, and does carry with it significant morbidity related to the surgery itself and potential complications, such as brachial plexus injury and shoulder drop.[48–50] Nonetheless, it certainly does open up a different aspect of tissue engineering and strategies for maxillofacial reconstruction.[51]

SUMMARY

Tissue engineering has come a long way in the last few years alone in terms of reconstruction of vertical alveolar ridge defects. The ideal construct comprises the three basic components for tissue regeneration: (1) cells that differentiate into the necessary type of tissue one is trying to engineer, (2) signaling molecules or growth factors that guide the cells to the correct pathway, and (3) a scaffold or matrix on which the tissue can be formed. Over the years many different combinations of these three basic components have been studied in human and animal trials, and have been met with varying degrees of success. There is no question, however, that tissue engineering is the future in regards to maxillofacial bony

reconstructive surgery, and will continue to evolve as concepts and techniques continue to be refined through research and technology.

REFERENCES

1. Rocchietta I, Simion M. Vertical bone augmentation with an autogenous block or particles in combination with guided bone regeneration: a clinical and histological preliminary study in humans. Clin Implant Dent Relat Res 2016;18(1):19–29.
2. Panagiotis M. Classification of non-union. Injury 2005;36(Suppl 4):S30–7.
3. Phieffer LS. Delayed unions of the tibia. J Bone Joint Surg Am 2006;88(1):206–16.
4. Marx RE, Morales MJ. Morbidity in bone harvest in major jaw reconstruction: a randomized trial comparing the lateral anterior and posterior approaches to the ilium. J Oral Surg 1988;48:196–203.
5. Miloro M, Ghali G, Larsen P, et al. Bone grafting strategies for vertical alveolar augmentation. Peterson's principles oral maxillofacial surgery. 2nd edition. Chapter 12. Hamilton, Ontario: BC DECKER INC; 2004. p. 230.
6. Chiapasco M, Casentini P. Bone augmentation procedures in implant dentistry. Int J Oral Maxillofac Implants 2009;24(Suppl):237–59.
7. Chiapasco M, Zaniboni M, Boisco M. Augmentation procedures for the rehabilitation of deficient edentulous ridges with oral implants. Clin Oral Implants Res 2006;17(Suppl 2):136–59.
8. Att W, Bernhart J, Strub JR. Fixed rehabilitation of the edentulous maxilla: possibilities and clinical outcome. J Oral Maxillofac Surg 2009;67(11 Suppl):60–73.
9. O'Brien F. Biomaterials and scaffolds for tissue engineering. Mater Today 2011;14(3):88–95.
10. Atala A. Tissue engineering and regenerative medicine: concepts for clinical application. Rejuvenation Res 2004;7(1):15–31.
11. Marx RE, Armentano L. rhBMP-2/ACS grafts versus autogenous cancellous marrow grafts in large vertical defects of the maxilla: an unsponsored randomized open-label clinical trial. Int J Oral Maxillofac Implants 2013;28:e243–51.
12. Kalfas IH. Principles of bone healing. Neurosurg Focus 2001;10(4):E1.
13. Wang EA, Rosen V, D'Alessandro JS. Recombinant human bone morphogenetic protein induces bone formation. Proc Natl Acad Sci U S A 1990;87:2220.
14. Yasko AW, Lane JM, Fellinger EJ. The healing of segmental bone defects, induced by recombinant human bone morphogenetic protein (rhBMP-2). A radiographic, histological, and biomechanical study in rats. J Bone Joint Surg Am 1992;74:659.
15. Reddi AH. Role of morphogenetic proteins in skeletal tissue engineering and regeneration. Nat Biotechnol 1998;16(3):247–52.

16. Hughes FJ, Turner W. Effects of growth factors and cytokines on osteoblast differentiation. Periodontol 2000 2006;41:48–72.

17. Urist MR. Bone: formation by autoinduction. Science 1965;150:893.

18. Bentz H, Nathan RM, Rosen DM. Purification and characterization of a unique osteoinductive factor from bovine bone. J Biol Chem 1989;264:20805.

19. Wozney JM. Overview of bone morphogenetic proteins. Spine 2002;27:S2.

20. Babensee JE, McIntire LV, Mikos AG. Growth factors delivery for tissue engineering. Pharm Res 2000; 17:497.

21. Uludag H, Gao T, Porter TJ. Delivery system for BMPs: factors contributing to protein retention at an application site. J Bone Joint Surg Am 2001;83-A(Suppl 1):S128.

22. Katanec D. Use of rhBMP2 in alveolar ridge augmentation. Coll Antropol 2014;38(1):325–30.

23. Wolff J. Das Gesetz der Transformation der Knochen. Berlin, Germany: Pro Business; 1892.

24. Tripplet G, Marx RE, Spagnoli D. Pivotal, randomized, parallel evaluation of recombinant human bone morphogenetic protein-2/absorbable collagen sponge and autogenous bone graft for maxillary sinus floor augmentation. J Oral Maxillofac Surg 2009; 67:1947–60.

25. Boyne PJ, Lilly LC, Marx RE. De novo bone induction by recombinant human bone morphogenetic protein-2 (rhBMP-2) in maxillary sinus floor augmentation. J Oral Maxillofac Surg 2005;63:1693.

26. Fahmy R, Mahmoud N, Cunningham L. Acceleration of alveolar ridge augmentation using a low dose of recombinant human bone morphogenetic protein-2 loaded on a resorbable bioactive ceramic. J Oral Maxillofac Surg 2015;73(12):2257–72.

27. El-Ghannam A, Cunningham L Jr, Pienkowski D. Bone engineering of rabbit ulna. J Oral Maxillofac Surg 2007;65:1495.

28. El-Ghannam A, Ning CQ. Effect of bioactive ceramic dissolution on the mechanism of bone mineralization and guided tissue growth in vitro. J Biomed Mater Res A 2006;76:386.

29. Miyazaki M, Tsumura H. An update on bone substitutes for spinal fusion. Eur Spine J 2009;18(6): 783–99.

30. Sauerbier S, Stricker A, Kuschnierz J, et al. In vivo comparison of hard tissue regeneration with human mesenchymal stem cells processed with either the FICOLL method or the BMAC method. Tissue Eng Part C Methods 2010;16(2):215–23.

31. Ardjomandi N. In vivo comparison of hard tissue regeneration with ovine mesenchymal stem cells processed with either the FICOLL method or the BMAC method. J Craniomaxillofac Surg 2015; 43(7):1177–83.

32. Kadiyala S, Jaiswal N, Bruder SP. Culture-expanded, bone marrow-derived mesenchymal stem cells can regenerate a critical sized segmental bone defect. Tissue Eng 1997;3(2):173–85.

33. Arinzeh TL, Peter S, Archambault M. Allogeneic mesenchymal stem cells regenerate bone in a critical-sized canine segmental defect. J Bone Joint Surg Am 2003;85-A(10):1927–35.

34. Shayesteh YS, Khojasteh A. Sinus augmentation using human mesenchymal stem cells loaded into a beta-tricalcium phosphate/hydroxyapatite scaffold. Oral Surg Oral Med Oral Pathol Oral Radiol Endod 2008;106:203–9.

35. Ueda M, Yamada Y. Clinical case reports of injectable tissue-engineered bone for alveolar augmentation with simultaneous implant placement. Int J Periodontics Restorative Dent 2005; 25:129–37.

36. Misch CE. Dental implant prosthetics. St Louis, Missouri: Elsevier; 2015. p. 573–99.

37. Aziz SR, Najjar T. Management of the edentulous/atrophic mandibular fracture. Atlas Oral Maxillofac Surg Clin North Am 2009;17:75–9.

38. Madsen MJ, Haug RH, Christensen BS, et al. Management of atrophic mandible fractures. Oral Maxillofac Surg Clin North Am 2009;21:175–83, v.

39. Cawood JI, Howell RA. A classification of the edentulous jaws. Int J Oral Maxillofac Surg 1988; 17:232–6.

40. Marx RE, Shellenberger T, Wimsatt J, et al. Severely resorbed mandible: Predictable reconstruction with soft tissue matrix expansion (tent pole) grafts. J of Oral Maxillofac Surg 2002;60(8):878–88.

41. Giannobile W. Periodontal tissue regeneration by polypeptide growth factors and gene transfer. Tissue engineering: applications in maxillofacial surgery and periodontics. Chicago: Quintessence; 1999. p. 231–44.

42. Guze K, Arguello E. Growth factor-mediated vertical mandibular ridge augmentation: a case report. Int J Periodontics Restorative Dent 2013;33:611–7.

43. Simion M, Rochietta I. Vertical ridge augmentation by means of deproteinized bovine block and rhPDGF-BB: a histologic study in a dog model. Int J Periodontics Restorative Dent 2006; 26:415–23.

44. Simion M, Rochietta I. Vertical ridge augmentation using an equine block infused with recombinant human platelet-derived growth factor-BB. A histologic study in a canine model. Int J Periodontics Restorative Dent 2009;29:245–55.

45. Simion M, Rochietta I. Three-dimensional ridge augmentation with xenograft and recombinant human platelet-derived growth factor-DD in humans: report of two cases. Int J Periodontics Restorative Dent 2007;27:109–15.

46. Stephan EB. Platelet-derived growth factor enhancement of a mineral-collagen bone substitute. J Periodontol 2000;71:1887–92.

47. Warncke PH, Springer IN, Wiltfang J. Growth and transplantation of a custom vascularized bone graft in a man. Lancet 2004;364:766–70.

48. Meijer GJ, de Bruijn JD, Koole R, et al. Cell-based bone tissue engineering. PLoS Med 2007;4(2):e9.

49. Ong HS, Ji T. The pedicled latissimus dorsi myocutaneous flap in head and neck reconstruction. Oral Maxillofac Surg Clin North Am 2014;26(3):427–34.

50. Sabatier RE, Bakamjian VY. Transaxillary latissimus dorsi flap reconstruction in head and neck cancer. Limitations and refinements in 56 cases. Am J Surg 1985;150:427–34.

51. Melek LN. Tissue engineering in oral and maxillofacial reconstruction. Tanta Dental Journal 2015;12:211–23.

Emerging Biomaterials in Trauma

Kirollos E. Zakhary, DDS, MD, Jayini S. Thakker, DDS, MD*

KEYWORDS

- Amniotic mesenchymal stem cells • Osteosynthesis • Bicortical fixation • Biocompatible
- Resorbable • Scaffolds

KEY POINTS

- The goal of research in the field of biomaterials is to find replacement constructs that can replicate, both in form and function, any lost or missing native tissue.
- The ideal characteristics of such constructs must mimic native tissues regarding weight, density, strength, and modulus of elasticity, among many others.
- Autografts are currently the gold standard for the replacement of missing tissues, but the possibility of producing replacement tissues without having a patient incur discomfort from a donor site is a close reality.
- Biomaterials currently in use include titanium, silicones, porous polyethylene, polylactic acid, vicryl meshes, and hybrids of these and many other materials.

 Video content accompanies this article at http://www.oralmaxsurgery.theclinics.com.

INTRODUCTION

Injuries of the facial skeleton pose unique and complex challenges to the maxillofacial trauma surgeon. Over the past few decades, significant advances in biotechnology have provided materials and tools to more efficiently, predictably, and reliably reconstruct and rehabilitate patients who have suffered such injuries. Goals to restore form and function have been aided immensely by the advent of new and innovative biomaterials and clinicians should strive to be familiar with and incorporate these new technologies.

This article reviews the various biomaterials available for repair and reconstruction of most maxillofacial injuries. The more common/traditional materials used to repair each type of fracture as well as some of the newer options available are reviewed. Indications and benefits for the various options of materials commonly used for each type of fracture are discussed.

IDEAL MATERIAL CHARACTERISTICS

Biomaterials are generally categorized as either naturally occurring or synthetic. Naturally occurring materials include autogenous grafts, allografts, and xenografts. Alloplasts are generally synthetic materials (**Table 1**).

Potter and Ellis[1] established the ideal properties of biomaterials. First and foremost, they should be able to replicate native tissues – that is, they should take on the required shape and contour of the tissues they are meant to repair/reconstruct, and they should retain those features. They may either be prefabricated to fit a necessary dimension or possess the ability to be cut/shaped to these required contours. Furthermore, they should also ideally have similar weight and density, modulus of elasticity, and strength of the tissue they are replacing.[1–4] For example, titanium plates used for mandibular reconstruction are designed to bear the load of occlusal forces while having

Department of Oral and Maxillofacial Surgery, Loma Linda University School of Dentistry, 11092 Anderson Street, Loma Linda, CA 92350, USA
* Corresponding author.
E-mail address: jthakker@llu.edu

Oral Maxillofacial Surg Clin N Am 29 (2017) 51–62
http://dx.doi.org/10.1016/j.coms.2016.08.010
1042-3699/17/© 2016 Elsevier Inc. All rights reserved.

Table 1 Biomaterials commonly used in maxillofacial surgery				
Metals	**Calcium Ceramics**	**Polymers**	**Acellular Biologics**	**Bioengineered**
Stainless Steel	Hydroxyapatite	Silicone	Collagen	rhBMP
Cobalt-chromium	Hydroxyapatite	PMMA	Dermal allograft	Amnion
Titanium	cement	Nonresorbable		Chorion
Gold	Bioactive glasses	polyesters		rPDGF (Gem21)
	Tricalcium phosphate	Resorbable polyesters		
		Polyamides		
		Polyethylene		
		Cyanoacrylates		
		PTFE		

Abbreviations: PTFE, polytetrafluoroethylene; rPDGF, recombinant PDGF.

the ideal strength and hardness to avoid fatigue or failure. Second, they should be biocompatible, meaning they are chemically inert, are nonallergenic, are noncarcinogenic, and do not promote bacterial growth or infection. Last, they should have adequate ease of handling. Again, the operator must be able to adjust the contour and size of the material to the appropriate dimensions as well as have the ability to fixate or otherwise stabilize it in the native tissues. The ideal material should also be sterilizable without deformation.

Additionally, it should be designed to remain in place indefinitely unless it is resorbable yet also easily removable if necessary due to rejection, infection, and/or failure.[5] If the material is designed to be resorbable it should be completely resorbed by the body in an appropriate time frame with minimal adverse biological reaction (**Box 1**).

Additional properties that are preferable include low cost and availability and radiopacity for radiographic evaluation. There is no perfect material for every indication or every situation, but the authors select the materials based on their properties and their applicability in each individual scenario. The advent of newer biotechnology has refined and perfected many of the properties sought in an ideal biomaterial.

REDUCTION AND OSTEOSYNTHESIS OF FACIAL FACTURES

Although description of specific operative techniques for the repair of each injury is beyond the scope of this article, the material properties for reduction, fixation, and reconstruction after several different types of facial injuries, including but not limited to, orbital, frontal sinus, nasoorbitoethmoidal, zygomaticomaxillary complex, Le Fort, and mandible fractures, are discussed. The various materials available for bone and soft tissue grafting in the immediate and delayed stages are also discussed.

Orbital Fractures

Material selection in the repair of orbital trauma is unique for many reasons, predominantly due to the shape of the bony orbit. Additionally, size, contour, number of walls involved, and the capacity for immediate versus delayed repair have played a role in implant selection. For the ideal orbital material, the implant should be able to be cut, contoured, and sized with precision, because the orbital volume is limited. Furthermore, the material should be malleable and without memory but have enough rigidity to retain a desired shape and support orbital contents. Likewise, the ideal orbital material must allow for enough support to enable restoration of volume and proper globe projection while also being thin enough to avoid exophthalmos when placed beneath the globe and orbital soft tissues. The material must also have a smooth surface to avoid impingement or

Box 1 Ideal properties of biomaterials
Replicate native tissue contour
Similar density/modulus of elasticity
Strength/stabilizable
Biocompatible/inert
Noncarcinogenic
Ease of handling
Cost effective
Available
Radiopaque versus radiolucent
Sterilizable

entrapment. The surgeon, however, must also be able to stabilize the implant to prevent displacement. It is also preferable to have a material that allows the evacuation of fluid in cases of bleeding with hematoma formation.[1,6] The ideal material should also have a low risk of infection, with a minimum porosity of 100 μm, because bacteria may be as small as 1 μm but macrophages are up to 80 μm in diameter.[6,7] Thus a larger pore size allows for access of these cells to destroy the bacteria that may inhabit the implant surface.

Autogenous, Allografts, Xenografts

For years, autologous bone for repair of orbital fractures was considered the gold standard. With recent advances in biomaterial technology, however, autologous bone for orbital complex injuries has fallen out of favor due to the surgical site morbidity associated with harvesting, limited quantity available, and unreliable resorption of the bone grafts. Furthermore, homografts and xenografts have been reported with mixed results in the literature, predominantly due to the lack of reliable resorption rates (**Table 2**).

Unlike its bony counterpart, cartilaginous grafts do not undergo active remodeling, and, unless violated or infected, do not have a propensity for resorption. Lyophilized or freeze-dried cartilage, both autogenous and allograft, have been sparsely reported in the literature, with largely unfavorable results. Their flexible nature has made them unpopular regarding long-term stability and are thus not regarded as an ideal choice for orbital reconstruction. Similarly, lyophilized alloplastic fascia and muscle have been reported for the reconstruction of small defects; their limited applicability also makes them an unpopular choice for orbital trauma, mainly due to their lack of rigidity and less than ideal rate of resorption.[1]

Metals

In 1967, the introduction of titanium to facial reconstruction by Snell[8] revolutionized the field of maxillofacial trauma. Prior to this, Vitallium (an alloy of cobalt, chromium, and molybdenum) and stainless steel were the standard of care. The metals, however, were plagued with problems with corrosion and poor handling properties (**Table 3**). Thus, in the 1980s, titanium became the standard of care for reconstruction of the maxillofacial skeleton – decades after other surgical specialties had integrated this into practice.[8] Titanium, like many metals, exhibits mechanical properties desirable for internal rigid fixation, and, when combined with its degree of biocompatibility, makes it a favorable material for fixation (**Table 4**). Definitions of important mechanical properties of metals are outlined[9]:

- Tensile strength – measurement of force required to break a material in a pulling vector
- Shear stress – measurement of force required to break a material in a sliding type vector (ie, how much force required to "cut" the plate in half)
- Modulus of elasticity – measurement of force required to deform the material in a reversible manner
- Yield strength – measurement of force required to deform the material in an irreversible manner

Other alloplastic materials

Other implants available include hydroxyapatite, silicones, porous polyethylene, polytetrafluoroethylene, polylactic acid, vicryl mesh, polydioxanone, and gelatin film. Although bare titanium remains a popular choice in the repair of orbital floor fractures, recent advances in hybrid materials have further enhanced the management of such injuries. Specifically, the advent of porous polyethylene with reinforced titanium mesh has become a

Table 2
Comparison of bone available for grafting

Bone Type	Advantages	Disadvantages
Autogenous	Osteoinductive potential Nonallogenic	Limited supply Unpredictable resorption Donor site morbidity
Allograft	No donor site morbidity Availability Osteoconductive	Delayed incorporation Risk of disease transmission
Xenograft	No donor site morbidity Osteoconductive Relative cost	Delayed incorporation Risk of disease transmission Greater risk of infection

Table 3
Metals used in maxillofacial surgery

Metal	Advantages	Disadvantages
Stainless steel	Low cost	Corrosion Late-onset implant failure Radiographic scatter
Vitallium	Strength	Difficult to shape Radiographic scatter
Titanium	Inert/noncorrosive Malleable Minimal CT/MRI distortion	Costly

staple in repair of orbital injuries. Such implants have the advantage of strength and shape retention offered by titanium while the polyethylene provides a porous biocompatible surface that allows for tissue ingrowth along the undersurface while providing a barrier that prevents such ingrowth on the orbital surface, thereby preventing restriction of the contents of the globe during extraocular movements.[10] Furthermore, titanium offers the advantage of visibility on postoperative imaging with minimal scatter, making the utilization of intraoperative CT a possibility; such technology has been shown to enhance the accuracy of repairs without significant increase in operative time.[11] Recently, the advent of patient-specific implantation (PSI) through preplanned thin-slice CT, particularly with polyether ether ketone (PEEK), polymethyl methacrylate (PMMA), and silicone implants, carries tremendous promise in the field of orbital as well as maxillofacial reconstruction (**Figs. 1** and **2**).[12] PSIs are manufactured to fit precise patient anatomy, through preplanned computer-aided design and computer-aided manufacturing. PEEK is a nonporous linear chain polymer exhibiting excellent strength and biocompatibility. PMMA is an inert synthetic polyacrylic resin also exhibiting excellent strength and biocompatibility, making both applications excellent for bony reconstruction.[12–14] Although the previous implants themselves are radiopaque, and thus subject to the same problems in postoperative radiographic identification as the other synthetic polymers, manufacturers are now adding barium to the polymer admixture to enhance radiographic identification, without compromise in function of the implant (Stryker, Kalamazoo, Michigan).

Frontal Sinus/Nasal Orbitoethmoidal Complex

Damage to the frontal and nasal orbitoethmoidal (NOE) complex provides unique challenges to the maxillofacial surgeon. The frontal bone not only houses the frontal sinus, which is lined by respiratory epithelium containing mucus-producing goblet cells, but also provides a major barrier from the intracranial compartment to the external environment. Likewise, the NOE complex is intimately associated with the bony orbit, because it contributes to the medial orbital wall as well as the nasofrontal duct apparatus. It is for these reasons that, beyond the traditional objectives of

Table 4
Titanium grades used in medicine

Grade	Composition	Tensile Strength (MPa)	Yield Strength (σ_y MPa)	Modulus of Elasticity (MPa)
1	Commercially pure titanium	240	170	102.7
2	Commercially pure titanium	345	275	102.7
3	Commercially pure titanium	450	380	103.4
4	Commercially pure titanium	550	485	104.1
5 (Ti-6Al-4V)	6% Aluminum, 4% vanadium	895–930	825–869	101–114
23 (Ti-6Al-4V ELI)	6% Aluminum, 4% vanadium Extralow interstitial	860–965	795–875	101–110

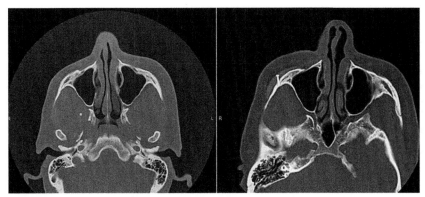

Fig. 1. This patient sustained a right zygomaticomaxillary fracture that was neglected for approximately 4 months and subsequently developed a malunion with evident deficiency in facial projection (*left*). To correct her post-traumatic deformity, secondary reconstruction with a custom silicone malar implant was undertaken (*right*). Note the improvement in soft tissue projection in the postoperative scan.

facial trauma repair, additional consideration into biomaterial selection is of paramount importance.

Anterior table

The anterior table of the frontal bone provides support and projection to the upper third of the facial skeleton, and, in the absence of a posterior frontal table, it is the protective layer of the neurocranium. Metals (predominantly titanium) are the mainstay of management of anterior table fractures and come in nearly limitless shapes and sizes. If the anterior table is amenable to open reduction, low-profile titanium plates and or mesh is the material of choice for internal fixation. In cases of avulsive defects,

autologous tissue transfer has historically remained the gold standard.[15–17] The realm of PSIs has, however, played a pivotal and revolutionizing role in the management of traumatic frontal and fronto-orbital reconstruction, with PEEK and PMMA the mainstay for custom modalities.[12,13]

Posterior table/nasofrontal outflow tract involvement

Management of posterior table injuries is rarely undergone with open reduction, but rather, the goals of treatment aim to prevent encroachment of the damaged bony particles on dura or frontal lobe tissue, which frequently involves removal of the

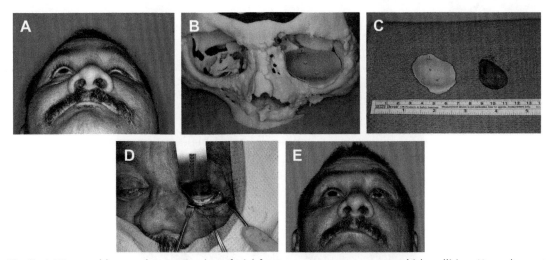

Fig. 2. A 50-year-old man who sustained panfacial fractures status post–motor vehicle collision. He underwent immediate rigid internal fixation of his facial fractures according to AO principles, with favorable results. Postoperatively, however, he required additional intervention for a residual enophthalmos (*A*) Preoperative enophthalmos. (*B*) Stereolithic model with custom PEEK implant. (*C*) Old left stock orbital implant removed; notice the size of the PEEK implant compared with the old stock implant in this large defect. (*D*) PEEK implant shown well-adapted to the orbit. (*E*) Postoperative improvement in enophthalmos.

posterior table (cranialization).[15,16] In the instance that function of the nasofrontal duct is compromised, options for materials for duct obstruction and sinus obliteration remain largely autogenous.[17,18] Muscle seems the most frequently chosen material for outflow obstruction, namely temporalis and tensor fascia lata, with or without associated fascia. If fascia is used alone, it undergoes substantial tissue shrinkage and greater volumes are needed for sustained outflow obstruction.[19] Alternatively, bone may be used for obstruction, especially if readily available. Options for obliteration of residual frontal sinus dead space include hydroxyapatite, glass wool, bone, cartilage, muscle, absorbable gelatin sponge, absorbable knitted fabric, acrylic, and fat, with fat the most popular choice. Fibrin tissue adhesives play a substantial role in the management of small cerebrospinal fluid (CSF) leakage and/or providing sealant properties after frontal sinus obliteration (Video 1; **Fig. 3**). Historically, 2 forms of fibrin adhesive were available: autologous and homologous donor fibrin tissue adhesives. Both operate as expected in vivo, promoting an

organized fibrin clot with strength from crosslinking. To date, autologous preparations have fallen out of favor due to the significant preparation time required perioperatively. Furthermore, comparative studies by Siedentop and colleagues[20] have shown that bond strength is markedly better in homologous preparations.[20] Disadvantages to using homologous preparations include risk of viral transmission, though this is extremely rare and a theoretic risk of Creutzfeldt-Jakob disease transmission.[20] Tisseel (Baxter International, Illinois, Deerfield) is a dual-component sealant containing human fibrinogen and aprotinin, which is activated by combining the human thrombin and calcium chloride component; the product is currently approved for any surgical application in which an adjunct to suture ligation is required to improve hemostasis and/or provide a barrier effect. Beriplast (CSL Behring, King of Prussia, Pennsylvania) is also a dual-component product consisting of a fibrinogen–factor XIII lyophilisate reconstituted with an aprotinin solution and a thrombin-calcium chloride solution that, when mixed together, activate to

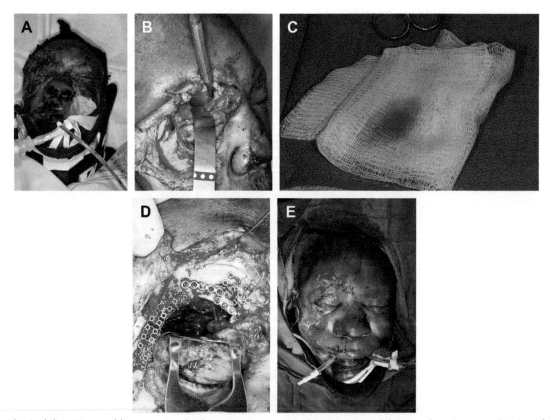

Fig. 3. (*A*) A 40-year-old woman involved in an auto versus pedestrian injury. (*B*) On exploration, an orbital roof fracture with pulsatile CSF leak was noted. (*C*) Positive halo sign for CSF leak. (*D*) CSF leak ameliorated with fibrin glue and bovine pericardium patch. (*E*) Immediate postoperative condition.

become a sealant similar to Tisseel (See **Fig. 3**). Both have been successfully used for repair of minor to moderate CSF rhinorrhea in the setting of frontal and/or NOE trauma as well as an adjunct to the frontal sinus obliteration/outflow obstruction techniques with desirable results.[21]

Midface

In 1901, the famous cadaver experiments by French surgeon, René Le Fort[22] popularized the midface fracture classification system still in use today. To date, treatment of midface trauma aims to reestablish the esthetic projection of the midfacial skeleton as well as provide a functional maxilla that relates to its counterpart, the mandible. Principles of maxillary traumatic deformities aim to reduce bony segments to premorbid alignment, largely through the use of low-profile titanium plates and screws. The prospects of titanium fixation cannot be discussed without addressing the characteristics of titanium used in the facial skeleton. **Table 4** describes the different types of titanium used in medicine and their relative advantages. Currently a vast majority of maxillofacial applications use grades 5 and 23 due to their superior strength, fracture resistance, and osseointegration potential.[23]

New to the arena of internal fixation of the craniofacial skeleton is the concept of resorbable plating platforms, which are predominantly indicated in the pediatric population. Potential advantages of resorbable plates include minimization of growth restriction, elimination of the need for delayed retrieval, superior imaging compatibility, and potential for avoidance of growing tooth buds.[24,25] The principal material used to date is a polylactic acid moiety; both poly-L-lactate and poly-D-lactate have been used alone or in combination, a 70/30 or a 50/50 poly-D-lactate/poly-L-lactate seems the most commercially available formulation (KLS Martin, Jacksonville, Florida). Although inferior to titanium in terms of rigidity and mechanical sheer strength, animal as well as human studies have shown similar outcomes. Operative considerations differing from traditional titanium fixation require a heating device for malleability to adapt the resorbable plate to the bony segments.[24] Likewise, sites for resorbable screw implantation must be tapped prior to installation, adding the potential for additional clinician error as well as material failure. Furthermore, the plates are bulkier, do not possess memory in the event that further bending is desired, and carry a small, albeit present, risk of inflammatory reaction.[26,27] To further complicate matters, a 2009 Cochrane review of 53 studies comparing titanium versus resorbable plates for facial fractures failed to find sufficient evidence regarding the effectiveness of resorbable plates compared with titanium plates.[28] At the time of this writing, no randomized controlled clinical trial exists to answer such a question.

Mandible

In a retrospective institutional analysis by Bell in 2007,[29] mandibular injuries were present in greater than 13% of all trauma patients admitted to one institution in a 10-year period, not including isolated facial injury victims. As such, it is apparent the magnitude and frequency with which mandibular trauma occurs are not infrequent. Furthermore, formal training of oral and maxillofacial surgeons in pertinent fields of dentistry, including occlusion and dental anatomy, should make them the most proficient authority with regard to mandibular trauma. It is, therefore, prudent for surgeons involved in the treatment of mandibular trauma to familiarize themselves with the materials available at their disposal for such purposes. Historically, Barton[30] bandage techniques and interdental wire fixation[31] were the mainstay of treatment of mandible fractures. As discussed previously, the advent of internal rigid fixation, namely titanium fixation, revolutionized the field of maxillofacial trauma, and mandibular trauma was no exception. A detailed account of the various properties of locking versus nonlocking, load-sharing versus load-bearing, and bicortical versus monocortical fixation is beyond the scope of this article; however, the significance of titanium fixation, as well as resorbable fixation systems (discussed elsewhere in this issue), and how it relates to mandibular trauma, is important.

Additionally, unique scenarios in treatment of the mandibular trauma exist. A prime example of the constant need for an evolving knowledge in biomaterials pertains to treatment of the edentulous mandible. Older techniques, such as Gunning pplints, split rib graft stabilization,[32] and the original methods of internal rigid fixation of Luhr and colleagues,[33] although historic, paved the way for modern principles of edentulous mandibular fixation. Although a 2009 Cochrane review by Nasser and colleagues[34] failed to delineate a single effective approach to treatment of the edentulous atrophic mandible, several investigators have suggested management strategies with favorable results. Among them, Tiwana and colleagues[35–38] advocate autogenous bone grafting to the severely atrophic mandibular fracture, whereas others, including the authors' institution, have had positive results with bone morphogenetic protein (BMP)-2 (**Fig. 4**).

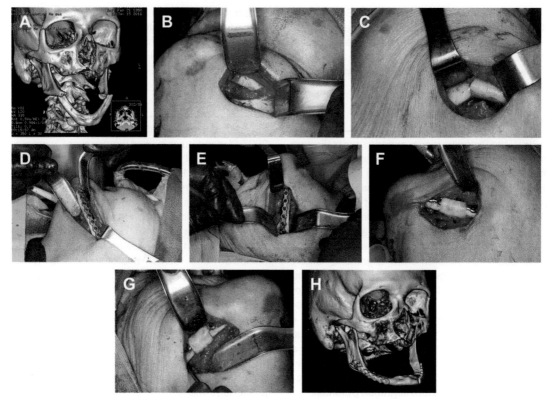

Fig. 4. (A) Preoperative atrophic edentulous mandible fracture. (B) Left body fracture prior to reduction. (C) Right body fracture prior to reduction. (D) Left body fracture postreduction and load-bearing plate fixation. (E) Right body fracture postreduction and load-bearing plate fixation. (F, G) Application of rhBMP-2 along *left* and *right* mandibular body fractures. (H) Postoperative radiograph (primary surgeon, A.S. Herford DDS, MD, FACS).

TISSUE ENGINEERING

Currently, the material of choice for the replacement of soft as well as hard tissue defects in maxillofacial trauma remains autologous tissue transfer, whether local, regional, or composite tissue transfer.[2] This is not without consequence, however, namely, donor site morbidity, prolonged hospitalization, and incurring cost associated with prolonged length of treatment. Recently, the advent of tissue engineering has become a vastly studied and rapidly expanding field of biomaterial science.[39] Benefits of bioengineered tissues include the amelioration of donor site morbidity as well as the capacity for the integrated tissue to mimic the native site to a degree not previously permitted by composite tissue transfer.[3,40] Currently, there is limited but promising application in the field of oral and maxillofacial trauma and reconstruction; to date, noteworthy applications in orofacial reconstruction have included bone, cartilage, fat, muscle, nerve, salivary gland, and dermal moieties, although preclinical trials may not successfully translate into clinically viable applications.[5,41] As discussed previously, for successful fabrication

and integration of bioengineered tissue to take place, 3 components are required: a scaffold capable of supporting the attachment, migration, and structural integrity of the bioengineered components; a progenitor cell lineage (ie, stem cell); and signaling molecules that stimulate stem cell induction and/or differentiation – this combination has been so-called the tissue engineering triad (**Fig. 5**).[3]

Scaffold

Arguably, the first step in a successfully bioengineered tissue begins with a proper scaffold. The scaffold itself provides an environment for the induction and/or conduction of the progenitor cell to form or create a functional tissue similar to that which it is meant to replace. For such events to occur, the scaffold requires the capacity for cell adhesion and migration and should possess the capacity to nurture growth and development without inhibition of the cellular proliferation process. Critical requirements for a biologically as well as mechanically viable scaffold include sufficient strength and rigidity to support the tissue in

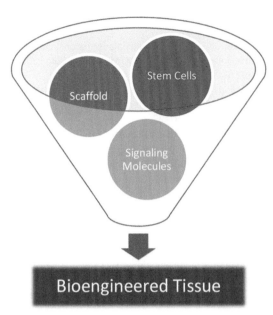

Fig. 5. Tissue engineering triad.

question, moldability/shapability, desired porosity for cell migration, desired surface properties to facilitate cellular adherence and delivery of nutrient requirements, and the ability to inhibit or avoid the host immune foreign body reaction.[4] Popular scaffolds include natural polymers (collagen, alginate, agarose, hyaluronic acid, silk, and chitosan), synthetic polymers (polylactic acid, polyglycolic acid, poly lactic-co-glycolic acid, and polycaprolactone), and ceramics (tricalcium phosphate, hydroxyapatite, and bioactive glass).[42–44]

Stem Cells

A stem cell, defined as a precursor cell that carries the capacity to differentiate into a specialized cell or a progenitor of various cells, may be used endogenously from the host or may be introduced from an exogenous source. For example, amniotic mesenchymal stem cells have been implanted into nasal defects in the New Zealand rabbit with statistically significant improvement in graft calcification as well as overall improvement in histologic organization of the implanted graft compared with the control arm.[45] To date, utilization of stem cells has largely been successful in the orthopedic and spine literature, namely with regard to bony regeneration. Stem cells currently under investigation with experimental as well as clinical use belong in 1 of 2 larger categories: adult-derived stem cells, which include popular applications of mesenchymal stem cells[44] and adipose-derived stem cells,[46] and the other category being human embryonic stem cells.[47]

Differentiation of the stem cell lineage into the appropriate functional unit not only is due to extrinsic signaling factors (discussed later) but also is largely influenced by the mechanical properties of the supporting scaffold.[44,48,49]

Signal Molecules

Perhaps the most successful molecular application available for use today in tissue engineering is recombinant human BMP (rhBMP), namely BMP-2 and BMP-7.[46,50] To date, clinical applications in oral and maxillofacial surgery with Food and Drug Administration approval is limited to sinus augmentation. The material has been used, however, in traumatic bony defects with largely favorable results.[50] Other signaling factors include vascular endothelial growth factor (VEGF), platelet-derived growth factor (PDGF), transforming growth factor (TGF), and fibroblastic growth factor (FGF), although in vitro applications to date have been limited.

With regard to applicability, 2 of the most common and successful applications in bioengineered maxillofacial reconstruction involve the use of BMP and PDGF. In his classic studies, to which there is still find applicability today, Boyne[50] found that the combination of a collagen scaffold with a BMP-2 signal molecule mixture in an osteoblast-rich environment provided an excellent medium for mandibular reconstruction of continuity defects. Furthermore, once reconstructed, such defects were rehabilitated with osseointegrated implants and exhibited favorable integration. Today, these concepts have been applied to the field of maxillofacial trauma with excellent clinical results. Furthermore, studies done on a PDGF-collagen combination show promising results for bony regeneration in the pig model, with applicability to human platforms.[51,52]

SUMMARY

Although cumbersome at times, an understanding of material science and emerging biomaterials for those treating maxillofacial trauma is an essential and ever-evolving facet of the surgeon's armamentarium. New and exciting technology in such a field is rapidly expanding as an era of demand for improved outcomes and less morbidity is entered. In particular, the arena of bioengineered tissue is making large strides in the forward direction of clinical applicability (**Box 2**). For instance, human amnion membranes for the use of traumatic bony exposure,[53,54] PDGF for bony defects,[51] and 3-D printing of scaffolds with precise control of repair biomechanics are all being avidly studied[4] and are expected to make positive

Box 2
Common tissue engineering components

Scaffold

Synthetic

    PLA

    PGA

    PLGA

    PCL

Natural

    Collagen

    Alginate

    Agarose

    Hyaluronic acid

    Silk

    Chitosan

Signaling Molecules

rBMP-2/7

FGF

IL

IGF

PDGF

TGF

VEGF

Stem Cells

Mesenchymal

Adipose

Epithelial

Endothelial

Chorion

Amnion

Abbreviations: IL, interleukin; IGF, insulinlike growth factor; PLA, polylactic acid; PGA, polyglycolic acid; PLGA, poly lactic-co-glycolic acid; PCL, polycaprolactone.

changes in the operative management of the trauma patient. Therefore, it is prudent for those involved in such trauma patients' care to seek an expanding knowledge base on the utility of emerging biomaterials.

SUPPLEMENTARY DATA

Supplementary data related to this article can be found online at http://dx.doi.org/10.1016/j.coms. 2016.08.010.

REFERENCES

1. Potter JK, Ellis E. Biomaterials for reconstruction of the internal orbit. J Oral Maxillofac Surg 2004; 62(10):1280–97.
2. Tevlin R, McArdle A, Atashroo D, et al. Biomaterials for craniofacial bone engineering. J Dent Res 2014;93(12):1187–95.
3. Ward BB, Brown SE, Krebsbach PH. Bioengineering strategies for regeneration of craniofacial bone: a review of emerging technologies. Oral Dis 2010; 16(8):709–16.
4. Moroni L, de Wijn JR, van Blitterswijk CA. Integrating novel technologies to fabricate smart scaffolds. J Biomater Sci Polym Ed 2008;19(5): 543–72.
5. Bhat S, Kumar A. Biomaterials and bioengineering tomorrow's healthcare. Biomatter 2013;3(3): e24717–12.
6. Ellis E, Messo E. Use of nonresorbable alloplastic implants for internal orbital reconstruction. J Oral Maxillofac Surg 2004;62(7):873–81.
7. Spector M, Harmon SL, Kreutner A. Characteristics of tissue growth into proplast and porous polyethylene implants in bone. J Biomed Mater Res 1979; 13(5):677–92.
8. Gilardino MS, Chen E, Bartlett SP. Choice of internal rigid fixation materials in the treatment of facial fractures. Craniomaxillofac Trauma Reconstr 2009;2(1): 49–60.
9. Niinomi M. Mechanical properties of biomedical titanium alloys. Mater Sci Eng A 1998;243(1–2): 231–6.
10. Sargent LA, Fulks KD. Reconstruction of internal orbital fractures with Vitallium mesh. Plast Reconstr Surg 1991;88(1):31–8.
11. Shaye DA, Tollefson TT, Strong EB. Use of intraoperative computed tomography for maxillofacial reconstructive surgery. JAMA Facial Plast Surg 2015; 17(2):113–9.
12. Kim M, Baohene K, Byrne P. Use of customized polyetheretherketone (PEEK) implants in the reconstruction of complex maxillofacial defects. Arch Facial Plast Surg 2009;11(1):53–7.
13. Frodel JL Jr. Computer-designed implants for frontoorbital defect reconstruction. Facial Plast Surg 2008; 24(1):22–34.
14. Owusu JA, Boahene K. Update of patient-specific maxillofacial implant. Curr Opin Otolaryngol Head Neck Surg 2015;23(4):261–4.
15. Bell RB, Dierks EJ, Brar P, et al. A protocol for the management of frontal sinus fractures emphasizing sinus preservation. J Oral Maxillofac Surg 2007; 65(5):825–39.
16. Rodriguez ED, Stanwix MG, Nam AJ, et al. Twenty-six-year experience treating frontal sinus fractures: a novel algorithm based on anatomical fracture

pattern and failure of conventional techniques. Plast Reconstr Surg 2008;122(6):1850–66.

17. Rohrich RJ, Hollier LH. Management of frontal sinus fractures. Changing concepts. Clin Plast Surg 1992; 19(1):219–32.

18. Fedok FG. Comprehensive management of nasoethmoid-orbital injuries. J Craniomaxillofac Trauma 1995;1(4):36–48.

19. Stanley RB Jr, Becker TS. Injuries of the nasofrontal orifices in frontal sinus fractures. Laryngoscope 1987;97(6):728–31.

20. Siedentop KH, Park JJ, Shah AN, et al. Safety and efficacy of currently available fibrin tissue adhesives. Am J Otolaryngol 2001;22(4):230–5.

21. Davis BR, Sandor GK. Use of fibrin glue in maxillofacial surgery. J Otolaryngol 1998;27(2): 107–12.

22. Le Fort R. Etude experimentale sur les fractures de la machoire superiore. Rev Chir 1901;23:208–27, 360–79, 479–507.

23. Elias CN, Lima JHC, Valiev R, et al. Biomedical applications of titanium and its alloys. J Minerals Met Mater Soc 2008;60(3):46–9.

24. Bell RB, Kindsfater CS. The use of biodegradable plates and screws to stabilize facial fractures. J Oral Maxillofac Surg 2006;64(1):31–9.

25. Orringer JS, Barcelona V, Buchman SR. Reasons for removal of rigid internal fixation devices in craniofacial surgery. J Craniofac Surg 1998; 9(1):40–4.

26. Boyette JR. Facial fractures in children. Otolaryngol Clin North Am 2014;47(5):747–61.

27. Siy RW, Brown RH, Koshy JC, et al. General management considerations in pediatric facial fractures. J Craniofac Surg 2011;22(4):1190–5.

28. Dorri M, Nasser M, Oliver R. Resorbable versus titanium plates for facial fractures. Cochrane Database Syst Rev 2009;(1):CD007158.

29. Bell RB. The role of oral and maxillofacial surgery in the trauma care center. J Oral Maxillofac Surg 2007; 65(12):2544–53.

30. Barton J. A systemic bandage for fractures of the lower jaw. Am Med Recorder Philia 1819;17:303.

31. Gilmer T. Fractures of the inferior maxilla. Ohio State J Dent Sci 1881-1882;1:309.

32. Obwegeser HL, Sailer HF. Another way of treating fractures of the atrophic edentulous mandible. J Maxillofac Surg 1973;1(4):213–21.

33. Luhr HG, Reidick T, Merten HA. Results of treatment of fractures of the atrophic edentulous mandible by compression plating: a retrospective evaluation of 84 consecutive cases. J Oral Maxillofac Surg 1996;54(3):250–4 [discussion: 254–5].

34. Nasser M, Fedorowicz Z, Ebadifar A. A Cochrane systematic review finds no reliable evidence for different management options for the fractured edentulous atrophic mandible. Gen Dent 2008; 56(4):356–62.

35. Tiwana PS, Abraham MS, Kushner GM, et al. Management of Atrophic Edentulous Mandibular Fractures: The Case for Primary Reconstruction With Immediate Bone Grafting. Journal of Oral and Maxillofacial Surgery 2009;67(4):882–7.

36. Van Sickels JE, Cunningham LL. Management of atrophic mandible fractures: are bone grafts necessary? J Oral Maxillofac Surg 2010;68(6):1392–5.

37. Carter TG, Brar PS, Tolas A, et al. Off-label use of recombinant human bone morphogenetic protein-2 (rhBMP-2) for reconstruction of mandibular bone defects in humans. J Oral Maxillofac Surg 2008;66(7): 1417–25.

38. Herford AS, Boyne PJ. Reconstruction of mandibular continuity defects with bone morphogenetic protein-2 (rhBMP-2). J Oral Maxillofac Surg 2008; 66(4):616–24.

39. Anderson JM. The future of biomedical materials. J Mater Sci Mater Med 2006;17(11):1025–8.

40. Rai R, Raval R, Khandeparker RV, et al. Tissue engineering: step ahead in maxillofacial reconstruction. J Int Oral Health 2015;7(9):138–42.

41. Bose S, Roy M, Bandyopadhyay A. Recent advances in bone tissue engineering scaffolds. Trends Biotechnol 2012;30(10):546–54.

42. Sherwood JK, Riley SL, Palazzolo R, et al. A three-dimensional osteochondral composite scaffold for articular cartilage repair. Biomaterials 2002;23(24): 4739–51.

43. Malda J, Woodfield TB, van der Vloodt F, et al. The effect of PEGT/PBT scaffold architecture on the composition of tissue engineered cartilage. Biomaterials 2005;26(1):63–72.

44. Engler AJ, Sen S, Sweeney HL, et al. Matrix elasticity directs stem cell lineage specification. Cell 2006; 126(4):677–89.

45. Turner CG, Klein JD, Gray FL, et al. Craniofacial repair with fetal bone grafts engineered from amniotic mesenchymal stem cells. J Surg Res 2012; 178(2):785–90.

46. Li W, Zheng Y, Zhao X, et al. Osteoinductive effects of free and immobilized bone forming peptide-1 on human adipose-derived stem cells. PLoS One 2016;11(3):e0150294.

47. Mele L, Vitiello PP, Tirino V, et al. Changing paradigms in cranio-facial regeneration: current and new strategies for the activation of endogenous stem cells. Front Physiol 2016;7:62.

48. Even-Ram S, Artym V, Yamada KM. Matrix control of stem cell fate. Cell 2006;126(4):645–7.

49. Guilak F, Cohen DM, Estes BT, et al. Control of stem cell fate by physical interactions with the extracellular matrix. Cell Stem Cell 2009;5(1): 17–26.

50. Boyne PJ. Animal studies of application of rhBMP-2 in maxillofacial reconstruction. Bone 1996;19(1 Suppl): 83s–92s.

51. Herford AS, Cicciù M. Bone resorption analysis of platelet-derived growth factor type BB application on collagen for bone grafts secured by titanium mesh over a pig jaw defect model. Natl J Maxillofac Surg 2012;3(2):172–9.

52. Herford AS, Lu M, Akin L, et al. Evaluation of a porcine matrix with and without platelet-derived growth factor for bone graft coverage in pigs. Int J Oral Maxillofac Implants 2012;27(6): 1351–8.

53. Tsuno H, Arai N, Sakai C, et al. Intraoral application of hyperdry amniotic membrane to surgically exposed bone surface. Oral Surg Oral Med Oral Pathol Oral Radiol 2014;117(2):e83–7.

54. Koob TJ, Lim JJ, Massee M, et al. Properties of dehydrated human amnion/chorion composite grafts: implications for wound repair and soft tissue regeneration. J Biomed Mater Res B Appl Biomater 2014; 102(6):1353–62.

Tissue Engineered Prevascularized Bone and Soft Tissue Flaps

F. Kurtis Kasper, PhD[a], James Melville, DDS[b],
Jonathan Shum, DDS, MD[b], Mark Wong, DDS[b],*,
Simon Young, DDS, MD, PhD[b]

KEYWORDS

- Maxillofacial reconstruction • Microvascular surgery • Tissue engineering • Bioreactors
- Growth factors • Personalized medicine

KEY POINTS

- Large composite defects of the maxillofacial region continue to pose major challenges to the reconstructive surgeon.
- Despite advances in reconstructive surgery using microvascular free flap techniques, donor site morbidity and the inability to recreate the original form of the bony defect has driven research into novel modalities of reconstruction.
- The in vivo bioreactor represents a promising method that combines microvascular surgical techniques with tissue engineering principles to create patient-specific vascularized bone flaps for the reconstruction of challenging maxillofacial defects.

INTRODUCTION

Large composite defects of the maxillofacial region pose major challenges to the reconstructive surgeon. This is especially true in the setting of a compromised wound environment (ie, osteoradionecrosis, contaminated/infected wounds, multiply operated sites). Advances in surgical techniques through the use of microvascular osteocutaneous flaps have increased the predictability of reconstructing large defects missing both hard and soft tissue. However, autologous tissue presents limited availability for transfer and is often not of ideal dimensions. Additionally, the harvesting of bone from the patient, either as a graft or as a free flap, necessitates donor site morbidity, with free tissue flaps requiring increased operating room time and technical expertise.

With the birth of tissue engineering in the mid-1980s[1] the groundwork was laid for identifying the different developmental processes and structures responsible for tissue and organ formation and applying this knowledge to regenerate tissue with anatomic accuracy and functional fidelity. Despite the transformation of tissue engineering from a nascent science into a scientific and commercial industry, few actual tissue engineering products have entered into clinical practice. One of the principal limitations identified by tissue engineers is the difficulty to create sufficient vascularity to support the constructs produced in the laboratory. This article describes the use of in vivo bioreactors to address this challenge and our experiences and those of others who have adopted this approach as a potential method of

Disclosure Statement: The authors have nothing to disclose.
[a] Department of Orthodontics, The University of Texas School of Dentistry, 7500 Cambridge Street, Suite 5130, Houston, TX 77054, USA; [b] Department of Oral and Maxillofacial Surgery, The University of Texas School of Dentistry, 7500 Cambridge Street, Suite 6510, Houston, TX 77054, USA
* Corresponding author.
E-mail address: Mark.E.Wong@uth.tmc.edu

producing composite grafts for maxillofacial reconstruction.

CURRENT METHODS OF MAXILLOFACIAL RECONSTRUCTION

Maxillofacial reconstruction has evolved from non-vascularized grafting to the introduction of microvascular free flaps in the late 1980s and early 1990s. The impact of free flap reconstructions has been so profound that it has been considered to be one of the most influential advances in head and neck surgery to date.

Generally, the goals for head and neck reconstruction are addressed with the use of flaps from one of three areas. The fibula, anterior lateral thigh (ALT), and radial forearm free flaps are the most commonly used donor sites because of their ease in harvest, modest donor site morbidity, and ability to include a large volume and variety of tissue types from a single vascular pedicle. For defects requiring composite soft tissue and bony reconstruction, options include the fibula, scapula, and deep circumflex iliac artery sites.

The fibula is commonly used for bony reconstructions of the head and neck because of its long bone stock, generous vascular pedicle caliber and length, ability to incorporate soft tissue, and acceptable morbidity at the donor site. Variations in anatomy of the fibula can limit the height and width of the flap requiring additional bone grafting procedures, and variations in the vasculature of the lower leg can affect the pedicle length necessitating the use of interpositional vein grafting. The lack of adequate bone height, especially when reconstructing nondentate mandibles, leads to discrepancies in the bone level and this can make dental rehabilitation a challenge. **Fig. 1** demonstrates a reconstructed

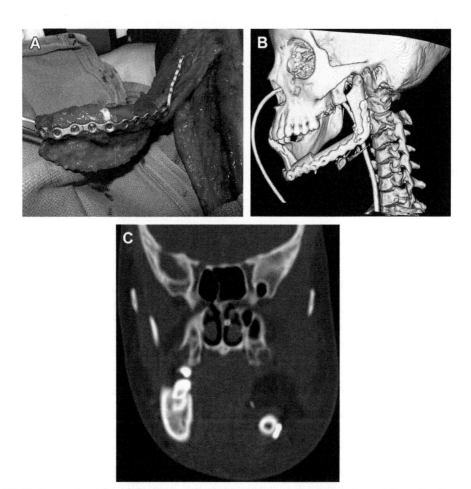

Fig. 1. (*A*) Fibular construct for a left segmental mandibulectomy defect before harvest from the donor site. (*B*) Lateral postsurgery three-dimensional reconstruction with fibular construct inset into recipient site of left segmental mandibulectomy defect. Note the deficient bone height compared with the contralateral mandible. (*C*) Coronal view at the level of the body of the mandible. The right native mandible is compared with the left reconstructed mandible.

mandibular defect with functional continuity; however, with a deficient fibular neomandible height. This is a common scenario that compromises the prosthetic reconstruction of the patient. The scapula is no better in terms of bone bulk, and possesses a shorter vascular pedicle, and the deep circumflex iliac artery bone flap has adequate bone but leaves a significant defect in the hip and is bulky and difficult to inset if soft tissue and a skin paddle is included. Although the success of microvascular reconstruction nears 95% to 100%, the quality of the reconstruction in terms of reestablishing the original form of the bony defect, preparation for dental rehabilitation, and need for subsequent revision surgeries leaves current microvascular techniques with room for improvement.[2,3]

TISSUE ENGINEERING APPROACHES

The limitations associated with current bone grafting options have stimulated the development of additional methods to augment bone repair, especially in more challenging defects. Tissue engineering strategies have emerged in recent years as a potential avenue to enhance bone formation in large defects while minimizing the morbidity associated with the use of autologous tissues.[1] Three tissue engineering approaches to create maxillofacial bone exist: (1) implantation of a scaffold that is conducive to bone tissue infiltration, (2) supplementation of a scaffold with bioactive molecules, and (3) implantation of cells in combination with a scaffold. Some approaches involve combinations of the various strategies to regenerate bone tissue, which increases the complexity of the technology and the associated regulatory burden for clinical translation.[2]

Once a construct composed of a scaffold, cells, and morphogens has been created, it has to be nourished during its early life. This is usually accomplished by placing the constructs within a device known as a bioreactor. Traditional in vitro bioreactors attempt to replicate outside the body key features of the in vivo environment to promote and support formation of three-dimensional tissue constructs tailored to meet the demands of the recipient site. A large variety of in vitro bioreactor systems have been explored for tissue engineering applications, and they generally provide mechanisms for controlling select environmental conditions, such as nutrient transport, mechanical stimulation, and oxygen tension, over the duration of culture. For example, some in vitro bioreactor systems are capable of overcoming the diffusional limitations for nutrient transport associated with traditional static culture techniques by circulating the culture medium through or around the three-dimensional tissue construct. By improving culture media circulation and convective transport of nutrients to cultured cells while concurrently providing mechanical stimulation to cells through fluid shear stress, such in vitro bioreactors are able to promote proliferation, differentiation, and uniform cell distribution on three-dimensional scaffolds.[3]

Although traditional in vitro bioreactor approaches have attempted to grow bonelike tissue in the laboratory setting, they are currently unable to recapitulate the complex microenvironment necessary to simultaneously form a vascular network.[4] There are reports of seeding clinically relevant (10 mL) volumes of ceramic particles with bone marrow stromal cells in perfusion bioreactors,[5] but the goal of growing bone constructs of a specific shape and clinically relevant size that can be transferred from a traditional bioreactor and implanted into a host recipient site remains elusive.[6] Additional studies have explored leverage of three-dimensional printing technologies for the fabrication of custom contoured scaffolds and associated bioreactors to support tissue construct formation in vitro,[7–9] yet vascularization of the constructs remains a critical challenge.

THE IN VIVO BIOREACTOR

To address these shortcomings alternative strategies, such as the in vivo bioreactor, leverage the innate potential of the body to generate vascularized bone tissue of a desired shape and size within an implanted chamber. The use of injectable hydrogels has been attempted for this purpose by injecting the material underneath the periosteum in a rabbit model,[10] but this approach lacks control over the final shape of the generated tissue, which is critical for reconstruction of facial bony structures. Similarly, although in vivo bioreactor chambers made of biodegradable polymers have been reported,[11] they are unable to maintain their predefined shape during the implantation period, suggesting chambers should be made of nonbiodegradable materials. Thus, to achieve improved geometric precision of the final vascularized bone construct, a nondegradable custom-shaped chamber can be filled with either osteoconductive or osteoinductive materials and then surgically implanted into a site remote from the recipient defect. Vascularized autogenous bone conforming to the geometry of the chamber is generated over a period of weeks, harvested with a vascular pedicle, and transferred to the bony defect for reconstruction and microvascular anastomosis.

The initial preclinical studies for evaluating this particular in vivo bioreactor strategy were carried out in a sheep model.[12,13] Rectangular chambers of polymethyl methacrylate (PMMA) were prefabricated in the laboratory with an open base, then filled at the time of surgery with morselized bone graft, porous poly(lactic-co-glycolic acid) wafers, or both and implanted in apposition to the osteogenic cambium layer of the rib periosteum (**Fig. 2**). After 6 to 13 weeks of implantation, the chambers were removed for histologic analysis, which demonstrated the generation of vascularized bone approximating the shape of the implanted chambers. Importantly, it was shown that the bone tissue could be removed from the chamber attached to vascularized periosteum with a vascular pedicle derived from the intercostal artery and vein (**Fig. 3**).[13] Collectively, these two proof-of-concept studies established the in vivo bioreactor approach as a promising method to generate vascularized bone of relevant size and shape. In keeping with the tissue engineering paradigm of optimizing combinations of cells, bioactive factors, and/or biomaterial scaffolds, additional investigations have studied different types of scaffold materials placed within the

in vivo bioreactor, and also examined the effect of various implantation durations on tissue formation within the chambers. An early study compared the use of poly(lactic-co-glycolic acid) wafers with or without the addition of autologous morcellized bone graft and found that new bone formation was only seen in areas that had originally contained the autologous bone graft. This illustrated that endogenous growth factors in combination with osteogenic cells and a mineralized substrate could enhance the performance of biologically inert biomaterials in this system.[12] Further investigations filled the PMMA chamber with either morcellized bone graft or autoclaved morcellized bone graft (thus inactivating any bioactive components including cells and growth factors) and implanted it in the sheep rib model for 3 to 24 weeks.[14] As expected, the chambers filled with native autologous bone showed optimal bone formation, whereas the groups treated with the "deactivated" bone graft yielded less bone tissue, likely because of a lack of osteogenic or osteoinductive cues (essentially mimicking a porous, degradable osteoconductive scaffold). Aside from studies that have characterized the effect of placing different osteogenic materials within the in vivo bioreactor, host

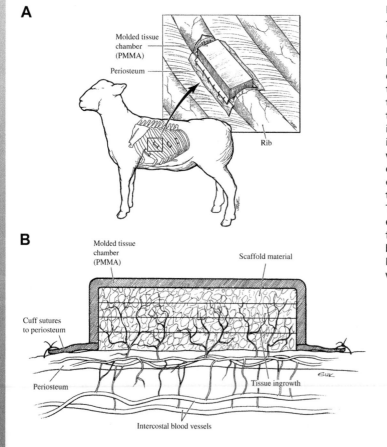

A

Molded tissue chamber (PMMA)

Periosteum

Rib

B

Molded tissue chamber (PMMA)

Scaffold material

Cuff sutures to periosteum

Periosteum

Tissue ingrowth

Intercostal blood vessels

Fig. 2. Sheep rib periosteum model for testing the in vivo bioreactor. (*A*) Up to four alternating ribs segments are removed and replaced by a nonresorbable bone-forming chamber with the open side facing the cambium layer of the rib periosteum. (*B*) Cross-sectional schematic through the long-axis of the in vivo bioreactor. Scaffold material is seen within the chamber with vascularization and tissue ingrowth occurring through the open face of the chamber in apposition to the periosteum. (*Adapted from* Thomson RC, Mikos AG, Beahm E, et al. Guided tissue fabrication from periosteum using preformed biodegradable polymer scaffolds. Biomaterials 1999;20(21):2007–18; with permission.)

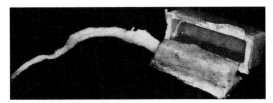

Fig. 3. Prevascularized bone flap formed by in vivo bioreactor chamber that had been placed in the sheep rib periosteum model for 6 weeks. (*From* Miller MJ, Goldberg DP, Yasko AW, et al. Guided bone growth in sheep: a model for tissue-engineered bone flaps. Tissue Eng 1996;2(1):51–9; with permission.)

variables, such as chamber implantation duration, have also been considered. For example, in the sheep rib periosteum model,[14,15] the duration of implantation was found to have a significant impact on the generation of bone. Optimal quantity and quality of ossified tissue was observed within a specific time window of 6 to 9 weeks, after which significant decreases in total bone volume occur. The reason for this is unknown. Another important host factor that has been shown to affect the generation of ossified tissue is the prefabrication site (ie, where the bioreactor chamber is implanted). Much of the initial preclinical work in the area of prevascularized bone flaps has used orthotopic sites, such as the sheep rib periosteum model.[12–15] However, several ectopic sites have also been tried using the in vivo bioreactor approach, with variable results. Chambers filled with morcellized bone graft implanted within the fascia of the latissimus dorsi muscle in sheep were found to generate primarily fibrovascular tissue (and exhibited significant graft resorption) in comparison with their orthotopically implanted counterparts.[16] Although this suggests that contact of the bioreactor contents with periosteum was more conducive to bone formation than contact with fascia in the muscle pouch, studies in small and large animal models have shown that bone formation in ectopic implantation sites is improved through the addition of exogenous osteoinductive growth factors.[17–19]

For recipient sites whose vascular bed has been significantly compromised, one potential benefit of the in vivo bioreactor approach is the ability to transfer a vascular pedicle, along with the bone flap. This approach was attempted in a pilot study using the sheep model[20]: PMMA chambers were filled with morcellized autologous bone graft, a ceramic synthetic bone graft material (85% beta-tricalcium phosphate/15% hydroxyapatite), or a combination of both and implanted in contact with the cambium layer of the rib periosteum for 9 weeks. Following this implantation period, these

prevascularized bone flaps were harvested with a vascular pedicle consisting of the intercostal artery and vein and used to reconstruct a 4 × 1 cm defect in the mandibular angle, with microvascular anastomosis to the vessels of the neck. These bone flaps remained viable for 3 months following reconstruction, and importantly, histologic analysis showed successful integration of the tissue-engineered bone into the native bone of the recipient site. Interestingly, the use of synthetic ceramic bone graft particles within the in vivo bioreactor did not seem to adversely affect the quantity or quality of bone generated within the chamber before harvest, as compared with the use of morcellized bone graft. This could have implications for future work by potentially decreasing the requirement for autologous bone harvesting, thereby reducing the donor site morbidity. However, being a pilot study, sample size was not sufficient to enable statistical comparisons, and further work is necessary to study the use of synthetic bone grafts for the generation of prevascularized bone flaps using the in vivo bioreactor approach. As the approach continues to be refined, emerging advances in three-dimensional printing technologies may be leveraged to enable the fabrication and use of patient-specific chambers tailored to the shape of the defect.

CLINICAL CASE REPORTS USING PREVASCULARIZED FLAPS

The face is synonymous with the person and reconstruction must attempt to restore form, function, and cosmesis. The ability to produce a customized vascularized flap that accurately replaces missing tissue will help fulfill these goals.

Currently five different prefabricated vascularized free flap approaches in human patients for mandibular reconstruction have been reported in literature.[21] The first case was reported by Orringer and coworkers[22] in 1999, and described a 52-year-old woman who presented with an angle-to-angle mandibular defect from a recurrent ameloblastoma. Reconstructive evaluation included bilateral lower extremity angiography that identified peroneus magnus (dominant peroneal vascular supply to the foot), a contraindication for free fibula transfer. Both iliac crests were previously harvested for mandibular reconstruction, which ruled out these donor sites. The authors used a Dacron-polyurethane tray shaped like a mandible, packed with autologous bone graft and exogenous growth factor (bone morphogenic protein [BMP]), which was placed under the dorsal fascia caudal to the right scapula. The graft was harvested 4 months later with overlying skin and encompassing fascia. The suprascapular vascular system was used as its pedicle. The pre-vascularized flap transfer was successful and the composite mandibular-chin defect was repaired. However, the patient was not able to tolerate oral feedings and dental implants were not placed because of lack of bone. The patient had multiple revision surgeries but ultimately passed away 2 years later because of disseminated disease of an unspecified nature.

Warnke and colleagues[23] described the next case in 2004 involving a 56-year-old man who had a titanium plate-only reconstruction for a body-to-body mandibular defect as a result of ablative tumor surgery 8 years prior. The patient also received 66 Gy of external beam radiation to the region. In this case, a titanium mesh cage was fabricated with computer-aided design and filled with bone mineral blocks additionally infil-trated with 7 mg of recombinant human BMP-7 and 20 mL of the patient's bone marrow. The construct was then implanted into the latissimus dorsi muscle for 7 weeks, and later transplanted as a composite tissue engineered bone and muscle free flap to repair the mandibular defect. Their technique involved harvesting a latissumus dorsi flap using the thoracodorsal/subscapular vascular system as the pedicle, which was ulti-mately anastomosed to the external carotid artery. Skeletal scintigraphy was used to deter-mine bone formation and remodeling within the in vivo bioreactor before the harvest. After 7 weeks, the prefabricated flap was harvested and transferred along with the encasing titanium mesh. Scintigraphy was once again used after transfer to monitor bone remodeling. The authors reported a successful result with restored es-thetics and function as the patient regained the capacity to enjoy solid foods. Unfortunately, after 13 months, the titanium mesh fractured, and the mucosa overlying the prefabricated flap dehisced resulting in bone exposure and subsequent infec-tion and resorption of the osseous component of the flap. Two subsequent revisions were per-formed, and eventually the patient died as a result of cardiac arrest.

In 2006 Cheng and colleagues[24] devised a mandibular ridge augmentation using a graft with an in vivo bioreactor approach. Unlike the previous reports, the authors in this study prefabricated a bone graft without a pedicle blood supply. The tis-sue engineered flap strictly relied on the perios-teum to revascularize by inosculation. The report detailed a 58-year-old man with a previous history of multiple flaps including a free fibula reconstruc-tion for buccal squamous cell carcinoma. The fib-ula was determined to be inadequate for dental implant placement. The authors used a PMMA chamber filled with harvested autograft and implanted it against the periosteum of the iliac crest. After 8 weeks, the tissue was harvested, and donor periosteum was sutured to mandibular periosteum to re-establish a blood supply. The pa-tient eventually died of hepatocellular carcinoma, but the authors note the transferred tissue was functional and retained three dental implants at 16 months.

Heliotis and colleagues[25] in 2006 planned a case avoiding autogenous bone harvest and main-taining an axial blood supply by implanting hy-droxyapatite blocks impregnated with BMP-7 into the pectoralis major muscle of a patient who had suffered from oral squamous cell carcinoma. After 3.5 months, bone scintigraphy revealed bone formation in the construct. The composite pectoralis major flap was harvested 6.5 months af-ter implantation and was successfully fixated to the recipient mandible with wires and an external fixator. Because of the bulk of the pedicle the au-thors did not tunnel the muscle pedicle but rather skin grafted it. After 4 weeks the pedicle was divided and the external fixator was removed. Although there is no radiographic study in the article to confirm bone union, the author noted they clinically felt a union between the bone seg-ments. Unlike previous studies, a biopsy was taken from the tissue at the time of transfer. The bone biopsy consisted of 17% bone, 37% hy-droxyapatite, and 46% fibrovascular tissue. After 5 weeks, the transferred tissue became infected, and the entire flap was removed. This case is notable for its histologic analysis of prefabricated clinical tissue and the ability to generate bone us-ing bone substitute materials alone.[25]

A more recent case report by Kokemueller and colleagues[26] in 2010 identifies a 57-year-old man who had a continuity defect from chronic osteomyelitis. The patient was initially recon-structed with a titanium reconstruction plate alone but desired bone reconstruction. The authors implanted cylinders of beta-tricalcium phosphate loaded with bone marrow and morcellized autolo-gous bone graft from the iliac crest into the latissi-mus dorsi of the patient. After 6 months, these cylinders were harvested from the muscle without the vascular pedicle. The construct was then transplanted to the defect site. Angio–computed tomography was used before transfer to confirm vascularization of the cylinders. Additional iliac crest graft bone was used to fill in the voids be-tween the cylinders. The authors noted at 12 months that the reconstructed mandible was still viable. Although not a prevascularized flap with a vascular pedicle, the case demonstrated successful generation of bone using an in vivo bioreactor approach.

In summary, all bone grafts regenerated with the in vivo bioreactor strategy were maintained in their heterotopic sites for an average of 4 months. The incubation time until flap harvest ranged from as early as 7 weeks up to 6.5 months. All studies resulted in bone formation within the in vivo bioreactor chamber. However, two out of five mandibular reconstructions failed or otherwise required significant revision. Infection of the hardware was cited as the main cause of the failures and this may be avoided with resorbable chambers and the immediate vascularization of the flap through the incorporation of a pedicle.

With modern biotechnology and tissue engineering the concept of the in vivo bioreactor and prefabricated flap is promising. These cases demonstrate the potential of this emerging science in the application of head and neck reconstruction. The main challenges to its true application are the following: (1) formulating a consistent tissue engineered graft; (2) identifying an optimal in vivo bioreactor site with a predictable vascular pedicle; and (3) the ability of the prevascularized graft to form a bony union to the recipient site, demonstrating integration into the recipient site.

STRATEGIES FOR THE CREATION OF PREVASCULARIZED FLAPS

In vivo bioreactors use the body's ability to regenerate tissue within chambers embedded remotely from the defect site, thereby removing the necessity to replicate the complexity of natural physiologic mechanisms in an artificial laboratory environment.[21] **Fig. 4** illustrates the steps involved in the prefabrication of a reconstruction construct using an in vivo bioreactor.[21] This concept was first demonstrated by Khouri and colleagues[27] in which a bioreactor filled with osteogenic growth factors generated vascularized bone tissue with specific anatomic geometries in rats. The application of an in vivo bioreactor can create a construct that gives a surgeon greater control over the reconstructive outcome. The size, shape, and tissue type can be customized to the defect. In addition, the selection of an appropriate donor site can influence the length, caliber, and number of vessels for the microvascular reconstruction.

Several clinical reports of in vivo bioreactor technology for the reconstruction of mandibular defects have been described. Implantation sites included the latissimus dorsi and pectoralis major muscles, the subscapular region, and the iliac crest.[22-26] These sites were selected because of accessibility and their rich vascular supply to

Considerations in Designing In Vivo Mandibular Bioreactor Strategies

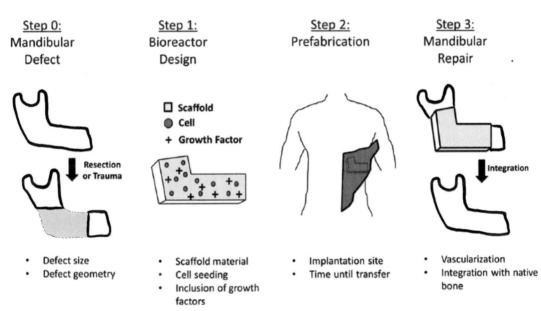

Fig. 4. Schematic demonstrating the general concept of the role of an in vivo bioreactor in the reconstruction of a mandibular defect. (*Adapted from* Tatara AM, Wong ME, Mikos AG. In vivo bioreactors for mandibular reconstruction. J Dent Res 2014;93(12):1196–202; with permission.)

nourish the planned neomandible. The desired site for bioreactor implantation should not cause significant morbidity, such as pain and inflammation, and it would be advantageous to select a site with suitable vessels for microsurgery.[13,21,28] For maxillofacial skeletal composite reconstructions, the selection of the prefabrication site is important because current studies suggest this directly affects the quality of the bone formed.[16] Placement of a bioreactor against periosteum has resulted in successful generation of ossified tissue, whereas ectopic growth of bone within soft tissue, such as muscle, has performed with limited success unless the bioreactor also contained exogenous growth factors.[17–19]

Animal studies demonstrate the ideal maturation time for bone in the setting of prefabrication for quality and quantity to be 6 to 9 weeks.[14,15] To maintain the shape of the prefabrication design, the bioreactor material should be constructed from nonbiodegradable materials.[11,21] To date, the optimal scaffold material within the bioreactor has yet to be determined and seems to have less significance than the location of the bioreactor against periosteum and/or the use of growth factors to be more predictable in bone growth.[14,19,29]

The combination of data acquired from animal studies, preliminary human reports, and current head and neck reconstructive trends would suggest to produce a vascularized bone flap, the ALT and fibula regions might be suitable as prefabrication sites. The ALT flap provides ample soft tissue components with the ability to include skin, fascia, and muscle based off of the descending branch of the circumflex artery. The vascular supply is suspect to several variations for the location of perforator vessels, which allows for the potential use of multiple soft tissue paddles. Current technologies, such as advanced fluorescence imaging to detect skin perforators, have become so accurate, that the design of the flap can be outlined before the visual identification of the perforator underneath the fascia. With this same technology, prefabrication at this site would be possible from a lateral dissection to expose the vastus lateralis and allow placement of the bioreactor without grossly violating the intermuscular septum between the vastus lateralis and the rectus femoris. The vastus lateralis muscle is supplied by perforating vessels to the skin and as such would be a choice donor bed for the placement of an in vivo bioreactor. It is one of four muscles that make up the quadriceps to extend the leg and can be completely harvested to an average dimension of 10 cm × 25 cm.[30] Although the vastus lateralis is the largest quadriceps muscle component and comprises 22% of the force exerted on knee

extension, studies suggest negligible donor site morbidity.[30,31] Multiple skin and soft tissue paddles would allow this site to compose variations for multisurface reconstructions of the jaw in addition to bone induction within a muscle and creation of a neomandible. **Fig. 5** demonstrates the exposure of the vastus lateralis in an ALT flap harvest that could be used as a site for prefabrication with an in vivo bioreactor.

The fibula free flap site should also be considered as a potential site because it is supplied with a consistent vascular pedicle and is easily accessible. Minimal morbidity and the potential for implantation of a bone chamber could occur without potential injury to the vascular supply.[32] In this scenario, the fibula can be accessed via a lateral approach to expose the anterior and lateral surface of the fibula, and because of the usual lack of height in the fibula for ideal mandibular reconstruction, the graft could be augmented by placement of a bioreactor construct along the surface of the fibula following a subperiosteal exposure. This area is already amenable to virtual surgical planning, and would allow for preparation and planning for the accurate placement of cutting guides and potential guides that act as an in vivo bioreactor. On average the bony segment of a fibula free flap can be 25 to 30 cm in length, with a skin paddle that can mirror the length and dimensions and encompass up to the entire surface of the posterior and lateral aspects of the lower leg. **Fig. 6** illustrates the potential use of an in vivo bioreactor at the fibula flap site. The use of virtual surgical planning allows for the accurate placement of the bioreactor to coincide with closing osteotomies to ensure an accurate alignment of the reconstructed mandible.

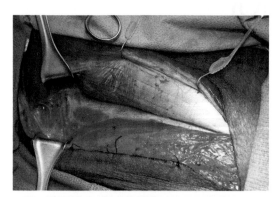

Fig. 5. This image demonstrates the ample muscle bed for in vivo bioreactor implantation in the ALT flap. The single asterisk denotes the vastus lateralis. The vascular pedicle is well visualized at the area denoted by the double asterisks.

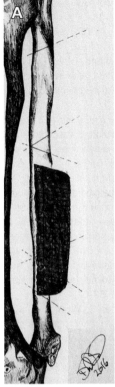

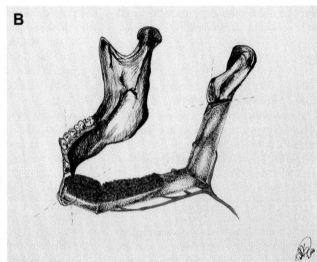

Fig. 6. (*A*) The fibula is visualized with the bioreactor aligned along the inferior third of the anterior lateral surface of the fibula. The bioreactor is depicted in this illustration in a *brown meshwork pattern*. The *red dashed lines* represent the location of the closing osteotomies to be performed to manipulate the fibula into the planned mandibular reconstruction. (*B*) The reconstructed mandible is illustrated with the left neomandible construct and the generated bone, *shaded brown*, from the bioreactor along the superior border to create an ideal bone height for dental rehabilitation.

The possibility of using virtual surgical planning to construct an in vivo bioreactor coinciding with areas that would augment deficient areas of the fibula for a more ideal neomandible bone height would resolve a significant limitation to this harvest site, as would the use of the ALT donor site to generate a prefabricated mandible within a rich vascularized vastus lateralis. Disadvantages associated with prefabrication include the additional surgery to place the construct to allow for maturation of the desired tissue. This may not be practical for cases that require immediate reconstruction. However, studies would need to be conducted to compare structural and functional outcomes with traditional means of microvascular reconstruction. By using favored microvascular reconstruction donor sites, we can optimize the quality of current trends for head and neck reconstruction.

Although not a microvascular flap, the use of a pectoralis major flap as an in vivo bioreactor is another novel approach the surgeon could use as a custom composite flap to reconstruct a mandibular defect. The approach would be similar to that described by Heliotis and colleagues[25] but would implant an allogenic bone construct with recombinant human BMP-2 and bone marrow aspirate in the most distal aspect of the flap instead of hydroxyapatite. Essentially, this would create a traditional pectoralis flap with a tissue-engineered bone in the muscle, and would rely on the thoracoacromial artery for vascular supply. The flap harvest and inset would be done similar to a traditional pectoralis flap, the only difference being that the proximal and distal ends of the bone would need to be exposed for osseointegration to the native mandible.

SUMMARY

The complex shapes of the skeletal components of the craniofacial region combined with the prominence of the face and paucity of overlying soft tissue create significant challenges for the reconstructive surgeon. In addition, the oral, nasal, and sinus cavities potentially expose grafts and flaps to contamination from secretions and organisms. Advances have been made with microvascular surgical techniques, tissue engineering of bone supplied with a vascular pedicle, and three-dimensional fabrication of implantable chambers customized to match a defect. By combining all these strategies, we hope to address several of the major problems associated with head and neck reconstruction and offer patients with facial defects a better reconstructive solution.

REFERENCES

1. Smith BT, Shum J, Wong M, et al. Bone tissue engineering challenges in oral & maxillofacial surgery. Engineering mineralized and load bearing tissues, vol. 881. Cham (Switzerland): Springer International Publishing; 2015. p. 57–78.
2. Atala A, Kasper FK, Mikos AG. Engineering complex tissues. Sci Transl Med 2012;4(160):160rv12.
3. Gaspar DA, Gomide V, Monteiro FJ. The role of perfusion bioreactors in bone tissue engineering. Biomatter 2012;2(4):167–75.
4. Liu Y, Chan JKY, Teoh S-H. Review of vascularised bone tissue-engineering strategies with a focus on co-culture systems. J Tissue Eng Regen Med 2015;9(2):85–105.
5. Janssen FW, Oostra J, Oorschot AV, et al. A perfusion bioreactor system capable of producing clinically relevant volumes of tissue-engineered bone: in vivo bone formation showing proof of concept. Biomaterials 2006;27(3):315–23.
6. Genova T, Munaron L, Carossa S, et al. Overcoming physical constraints in bone engineering: "the importance of being vascularized." J Biomater Appl 2015;30(7):940–51.
7. Temple JP, Yeager K, Bhumiratana S, et al. Bioreactor cultivation of anatomically shaped human bone grafts. Methods Mol Biol 2014;1202(Chapter 33):57–78.
8. Temple JP, Hutton DL, Hung BP, et al. Engineering anatomically shaped vascularized bone grafts with hASCs and 3D-printed PCL scaffolds. J Biomed Mater Res A 2014;102(12):4317–25.
9. Costa PF, Vaquette C, Baldwin J, et al. Biofabrication of customized bone grafts by combination of additive manufacturing and bioreactor knowhow. Biofabrication 2014;6(3):035006.
10. Stevens MM, Marini RP, Schaefer D, et al. In vivo engineering of organs: the bone bioreactor. Proc Natl Acad Sci U S A 2005;102(32):11450–5.
11. Warnke PH, Springer IN, Acil Y, et al. The mechanical integrity of in vivo engineered heterotopic bone. Biomaterials 2006;27(7):1081–7.
12. Thomson RC, Mikos AG, Beahm E, et al. Guided tissue fabrication from periosteum using preformed biodegradable polymer scaffolds. Biomaterials 1999;20(21):2007–18.
13. Miller MJ, Goldberg DP, Yasko AW, et al. Guided bone growth in sheep: a model for tissue-engineered bone flaps. Tissue Eng 1996;2(1):51–9.
14. Cheng M-H, Brey EM, Allori A, et al. Ovine model for engineering bone segments. Tissue Eng 2005; 11(1–2):214–25.
15. Cheng M-H, Brey EM, Allori AC, et al. Periosteum-guided prefabrication of vascularized bone of clinical shape and volume. Plast Reconstr Surg 2009; 124(3):787–95.
16. Brey EM, Cheng M-H, Allori A, et al. Comparison of guided bone formation from periosteum and muscle fascia. Plast Reconstr Surg 2007;119(4):1216–22.
17. Geuze RE, Theyse LFH, Kempen DHR, et al. A differential effect of bone morphogenetic protein-2 and vascular endothelial growth factor release timing on osteogenesis at ectopic and orthotopic sites in a large-animal model. Tissue Eng Part A 2012;18(19–20):2052–62.
18. Roldán JC, Jepsen S, Miller J, et al. Bone formation in the presence of platelet-rich plasma vs. bone morphogenetic protein-7. Bone 2004;34(1): 80–90.
19. Kusumoto K, Bessho K, Fujimura K, et al. Prefabricated muscle flap including bone induced by recombinant human bone morphogenetic protein-2: an experimental study of ectopic osteoinduction in a rat latissimus dorsi muscle flap. Br J Plast Surg 1998;51(4):275–80.
20. Tatara AM, Kretlow JD, Spicer PP, et al. Autologously generated tissue-engineered bone flaps for reconstruction of large mandibular defects in an ovine model. Tissue Eng Part A 2015;21(9–10):1520–8.
21. Tatara AM, Wong ME, Mikos AG. In vivo bioreactors for mandibular reconstruction. J Dent Res 2014; 93(12):1196–202.
22. Orringer JS, Shaw WW, Borud LJ, et al. Total mandibular and lower lip reconstruction with a prefabricated osteocutaneous free flap. Plast Reconstr Surg 1999;104(3):793–7.
23. Warnke PH, Springer ING, Springer ING, et al. Growth and transplantation of a custom vascularised bone graft in a man. Lancet 2004;364(9436): 766–70.
24. Cheng M-H, Brey EM, Ulusal BG, et al. Mandible augmentation for osseointegrated implants using tissue engineering strategies. Plast Reconstr Surg 2006;118(1):1e–4e.
25. Heliotis M, Lavery KM, Ripamonti U, et al. Transformation of a prefabricated hydroxyapatite/osteogenic protein-1 implant into a vascularised pedicled bone flap in the human chest. Int J Oral Maxillofac Surg 2006;35(3):265–9.
26. Kokemueller H, Spalthoff S, Nolff M, et al. Prefabrication of vascularized bioartificial bone grafts

in vivo for segmental mandibular reconstruction: experimental pilot study in sheep and first clinical application. Int J Oral Maxillofac Surg 2010;39(4): 379–87.

27. Khouri RK, Koudsi B, Reddi H. Tissue transformation into bone in vivo: a potential practical application. JAMA 1991;266(14):1953–5.

28. McCullen SD, Chow AG, Stevens MM. In vivo tissue engineering of musculoskeletal tissues. Curr Opin Biotechnol 2011;22(5):715–20.

29. Eweida AM, Nabawi AS, Marei MK, et al. Mandibular reconstruction using an axially vascularized tissue-

engineered construct. Ann Surg Innov Res 2011; 5(1):1.

30. Spyriounis PK, Lutz BS. Versatility of the free vastus lateralis muscle flap. J Trauma 2008;64(4):1100–5.

31. Narici MV, Landoni L, Minetti AE. Assessment of human knee extensor muscles stress from in vivo physiological cross-sectional area and strength measurements. Eur J Appl Physiol Occup Physiol 1992;65(5):438–44.

32. Shpitzer T, Neligan P, Boyd B, et al. Leg morbidity and function following fibular free flap harvest. Ann Plast Surg 1997;38(5):460–4.

Maxillofacial Defects and the Use of Growth Factors

Alan S. Herford, DDS, MD[a],*, Meagan Miller, DDS[a], Fabrizio Signorino, DDS[b]

KEYWORDS

- Maxillofacial defects • Regenerative medicine • Grafts • Growth factors • BMP

KEY POINTS

- Growth factors can be used in addition to or as an alternative to conventional reconstruction techniques for maxillofacial defects.
- Recombinant human bone morphogenic protein-2 has been shown to be the most promising among the growth factors, showing good results when applied in clinical studies.
- The clinical applications of growth factors may represent a solution or alternative to the need for donor sites and improve qualitative and quantitative bone healing.
- The lack of information concerning doses, indications, and/or adverse reactions and complications still limits the use of growth factors as routine treatment.

INTRODUCTION

Despite recent advances in regenerative medicine, reconstruction of maxillofacial defects remains a challenge. These challenges stem from the complex set of criteria that needs to be met for a successful substitute to restore, maintain, and improve tissue function. There are many causes of tissue loss, including trauma, pathologic processes, and congenital anomalies. The resulting characteristics such as the size, geometry, and vascularity of the defects dictate the surgical options available for treatment. Grafting of the defective site can be performed with different biomaterial options. Autologous bone grafts and free vascularized fibular grafts are considered to be the gold standard for treating these defects.[1]

Autogenous bone grafts have the advantage of stimulating bone regeneration through osteoinduction while avoiding an immunologic reaction. For large continuity defects, harvested iliac crest bone is used in conjunction with reconstruction plates. Continuity defects involving the removal of a malignancy will often result in both a hard and soft tissue defect that may best be treated with free tissue microvascular flaps.[2] These flaps can be suitable options for patients who are undergoing radiotherapy. Although holding a high success rate for reconstructing bone defects, the limitations surrounding the use of autogenous flaps arise from donor site morbidity and the variable quantity and quality of tissue harvested. The chosen donor site may not provide adequate bone graft material for the defect, depending on the size. Other adverse events include damage to adjacent structures, infection, and prolonged pain at the donor site. Bone grafting can have unpredictable resorption and difficulties in maintaining closure of the soft tissue over the graft.[3,4] Although they provide the most biocompatible option, the disadvantages of autogenous grafts have driven the search for alternatives.

Allogeneic bone grafts provide an attractive alternative option to regenerate bone defects. These types of bone grafts provide an osteoconductive scaffold for bone ingrowth without the

Disclosure Statement: The authors have nothing to disclose.
a Oral & Maxillofacial Surgery, Loma Linda University, 11092 Anderson Street, Loma Linda, CA 92350, USA;
b Oral Surgery, Department of Dental Implants, University of Milan, Via Commenda 10, Milan 20122, Italy
* Corresponding author.
E-mail address: aherford@llu.edu

associated morbidity of an autograft. A primary disadvantage of allograft bone as a graft option is the loss of the majority of its associated growth factors during the sterilization process.[5] The significant changes to its architecture allows for bone ingrowth from the perimeter of the defect rather than new bone formation de novo. To accomplish the regeneration of a bone defect, the bone margins must exceed the rate of fibrogenesis growing in from the surrounding soft tissue.[6] Because of the limitations of this type of graft, allografts may be successful in small defects but are rather limited for larger defects.

The surgeon must weigh the risks specific to autograft harvest versus the limited ability of bone regeneration associated with allograft materials when planning the reconstruction of maxillofacial defects. The addition of growth factors combined with various types of graft materials and techniques have shown to be a promising effort in the improvement of bone regeneration.

GROWTH FACTORS

Growth factors are defined as a group of proteins capable of stimulating cellular growth, migration, proliferation, and differentiation. These signaling molecules can generate different kinds of effects by upregulating or downregulating the synthesis of proteins and receptors.[7–9] The importance of the role of these molecules is well-recognized, even if all the mechanisms involved are not completely known. Growth factors are involved in tissue formation beginning in the embryologic phases. Mutations in the genes that code for these proteins can cause various craniofacial skeletal anomalies resulting in certain syndromes (ie, Apert syndrome, Crouzon syndrome, and the achondroplasia syndromes).[10]

With the advances in recombinant technology, growth factors and biologics have become available as an alternative to traditional grafting procedures. Growth factors have been used to augment bone formation with various grafting techniques. Several of these signaling molecules have been studied for their inductive regenerative potential such as vascular endothelial growth factor (VEGF), fibroblast growth factors (FGF), platelet-derived growth factor (PDGF), platelet rich Plasma (PRP), and bone morphogenic proteins (BMPs).[11,12]

VASCULAR ENDOTHELIAL GROWTH FACTOR

For proper healing to take place, the defect must have appropriate vascularization. Much of the formation and maintenance of angiogenesis is orchestrated by VEGF. It has been well-documented that VEGF, as a part of the cascade, controls bone development during the promotion of vascular structures, particularly in the process of bone healing, by acting on osteoblasts.[13–15] Just as blood vessel formation does not occur at 1 specific time, the deposition of 1 particular type of VEGF at a high concentration within a defect is not likely to produce a vasculature system. The release of VEGF over time and other confounding factors create a unique challenge in creating a vasculature that could support a regenerative tissue construct. A temporal formulation of VEGF, applied locally at the site of bone damage, may prove to be an effective therapy to promote human bone repair.[14,16] Zhang and colleagues[17] investigated the effects of VEGF alone and in association to BMP-2. They observed how the application of a single angiogenic agent was not sufficient for bone generation. However, the effect of VEGF simultaneously applied with BMP-2 enhanced the bone formation, in terms of both density and volume. Furthermore, VEGF was significantly effective in increasing the resorption speed of the carrier used in the study.

FIBROBLAST GROWTH FACTOR

The role of FGFs and their receptors in fracture healing has been widely analyzed and discussed. In small and large rodents and nonhuman primates, FGF2 has been found to stimulate the proliferation of periosteal cells, osteoprogenitors, and chondrogenitors, enhancing callus formation.[18] FGF application, with FGF2 above all, has been studied for promoting fracture healing. However, some studies showed that FGF2 treatment was not effective in increasing bone mineral density or mechanical strength of the callus.[19] This can be explained by suggesting that the effect of FGF on bone formation is biphasic, with inhibitory effects at high doses.[18] Kawaguchi and colleagues[20] showed instead how topical application of recombinant human FGF2 shortens the healing time of tibial shaft fracture, with a higher percentage of radiographic bone union. These papers suggest that FGFs' usefulness is not clearly demonstrated, however, a precise, time-controlled regulation of FGF signaling during bone healing may be helpful in bone-regenerative procedures, including those of the oral cavity.

PLATELET-DERIVED GROWTH FACTOR

PDGF has an active role in the wound healing processes of various tissues, including bone. The most important specific activities of PDGF include mitogenesis, angiogenesis, and macrophage activation. PDGF ligands and receptors have been detected in osteoblasts, chondrocytes, and mesenchymal stem cells.[21] When PDGF receptors α and β were removed in mice, it was observed that the primary effects of PDGF signaling in bone healing are proliferation and migration responses.[22] The use of PDGF in addition to a collagen matrix has been shown to accelerate soft tissue healing and promote bone formation.[23] Guven and colleagues observed how the association of PDGF and an absorbable collagen sponge (ACS) as a carrier, seems to be more effective in bone formation in the late healing period respect ACS and rhBMP-2.[24]

PLATELET-RICH PLASMA

Platelet-rich plasma is an autologous source of PDGF and transforming growth factor beta (TGF-β) that is obtained by sequestering and concentrating platelets by gradient density centrifugation. PRP increases platelet concentration when placed into grafts, showing the presence of at least 3 growth factors (PDGF, TGF-β1, and TGF-β2) and, sequentially, that cancellous marrow cells have receptors for these growth factors. The effects of the release of PDGF and TGF-β, from the degranulation of platelets in the graft, are related to the initial phase of bone regeneration. Some studies reported a positive effect in enhancing both soft and hard tissue healing,[25,26] whereas others did not show apparent benefit for either bone formation or implant survival rate.[27,28] Marx and colleagues[25] showed how the additional amounts of these growth factors obtained by adding platelet rich plasma to grafts evidenced a radiographic maturation rate 1.62 to 2.16 times that of grafts without platelet-rich plasma. It was also observed that a greater bone density was present in grafts in which platelet-rich plasma was added. Even if these data indicate promising results in the application of PRP, the literature was not able to confirm with conclusive evidence the advantage of the application of PRP in bone regeneration procedures.

BONE MORPHOGENIC PROTEIN

As discussed, many growth factors are involved in osteogenesis and during the early phases of fracture healing. Historically, Urist[29] in 1965 observed new local bone formation in rodents after they underwent intramuscular implantation of bone cylinders. This phenomenon was attributed to BMPs. BMPs recruit stem cells to the healing site and then differentiate them into the osteogenic lineage

for bone deposition. Currently, more than 20 BMPs have been discovered; however, only a few of them seem to be osteoinductive.[30] Specifically, BMP-2 and BMP-7 have been shown to play an important role in inducing bone formation for fracture repair.[31–33] Currently, the BMPs are grouped into the TGF-β superfamily because of their similarities in protein structure and sequence homology. The term transforming growth factor beta (TGF-β) is applied to the superfamily of growth and differentiating factors of which the bone morphogenetic protein family is a member. TGF-β1 and TGF-β2 proteins are involved with general connective tissue repair and bone regeneration.[34] These proteins are synthesized and found in platelets and macrophages as well as in some other cell types. In an active wound, they are released by platelet degranulation or actively secreted by macrophages and act as growth factors affecting mainly fibroblasts and marrow stem cells. TGF-β proteins therefore represent a mechanism for sustaining a long-term healing and bone regeneration module and may even evolve into a bone remodeling factor over time. They possess the ability to stimulate osteoblast deposition of the collagen matrix of wound healing and of bone.[34] The most important functions are chemotaxis and mitogenesis of osteoblast precursors. In addition, TGF-β factors inhibit osteoclast formation and bone resorption, thus favoring bone formation over resorption.

BMPs have been used as a therapeutic option in order to stimulate new bone formation.[35] Recombinant human BMP (rhBMP) in combination with a collagen sponge carrier made out of type 1 bovine collagen has been approved by the US Food and Drug Administration and is used for specific clinical situations, namely, interbody spinal fusion, open tibial fractures, sinus augmentation, and localized alveolar ridge augmentation after dental extraction. Other applications have been reported in the literature with various success rates. BMPs have been shown to successfully reconstruct defects ranging from isolated areas of the jaw to entire restoration of defects. An advantage of BMP is that a donor site is not required, thus reducing the time and potential morbidity associated with harvesting autogenous graft material.

BMPs are delivered to the recipient site as part of a surgical procedure via a carrier/delivery system, which may also provide limited mechanical support. These systems, which are absorbed over time, function to maintain the concentration of the BMP at the treatment site, providing temporary scaffolding for osteogenesis, and prevent extraneous bone formation or toxic events. Carrier systems have included inorganic material, synthetic polymer, natural polymers, and bone allograft. Carrier and delivery systems are important variables in the clinical use of BMP. The system consists of rhBMP-2 and an ACS as the carrier. BMP-2 is available as a lyophilized powder in vials containing the growth factor. After reconstitution with normal saline, the configuration results in a concentration of 1.5 mg/mL. The solution is then applied to the ACS provided and should be used after a minimum of 15 minutes to allow for the integration of the growth factor with the carrier. The ACS has been evaluated in numerous in vivo models and clinical trials and is the only carrier currently approved by the US Food and Drug Administration for clinical use. However, other carrier systems are being developed showing promising results in preclinical studies.[36–39]

In patients requiring staged maxillary sinus floor augmentation, rhBMP-2/ACS has been shown to safely induce adequate bone formation for the placement and functional loading of endosseous dental implants. The sponge regulates the slow release of BMP-2 and keeps the growth factor distribution in the defect area, preventing adverse toxic events. However, the ACS is compressible and does not ideally support soft tissues to maintain space for osteogenesis to occur. The concavity, walls, and floor of the sinus help to keep the ACS position over time.

Grafting with BMP is contraindicated in patients who are pregnant, may be allergic to any of the materials contained in the devices, have an infection near the area of the surgical incision, have had a tumor removed from the area of the implantation site or currently have a tumor in that area, or are skeletally immature. Few documented adverse events can be attributed to BMP. Nonetheless, any complications and safety issues are of concern. Adverse events that have been reported include but are not limited to immune responses, inflammation, ectopic bone formation, infection, vertebral osteolysis, and vertebral edema.

Currently, rhBMP-2 is approved for localized alveolar defects. Studies have shown that the use of BMP is useful in the enhancement of bone formation when used in conjunction with bone grafting procedures. This protein is combined with an ACS and induces bone formation through the recruitment and differentiation of mesenchymal stem cells.[40] BMPs may stimulate the expression of VEGF by osteoblasts[41]; however, Zhan and colleagues[17] showed that the neoangiogenesis achieved cannot be compared with the one obtained by the application of VEGF alone.

CLINICAL APPLICATION OF RECOMBINANT HUMAN BONE MORPHOGENIC PROTEIN-2

The clinical application of growth factors continues to evolve with the goal of improving the treatment of various types of alveolar defects. Several studies have shown encouraging clinical results using BMP-2 for reconstructing a variety of defects. Boyne and colleagues[42] demonstrated how mean bone height changes depending on the applied concentration. Comparing 0.75 and 1.5 mg/mL concentrations, it was shown how the higher bone level rates were associated with the second group in a sinus floor augmentation study model. After identifying 1.5 mg/mL of rhBMP-2 as the most effective concentration, a randomized, multicenter, pilot study was performed examining the safety and efficacy of INFUSE Bone Graft (Medtronic, Minneapolis, MN) in sinus floor augmentations.[43] A total of 160 patients were treated with 1.5 mg/mL rhBMP-2/ACS (n = 82) or bone graft (n = 78). The bone graft group consisted of autogenous bone alone or in combination with allogeneic bone. The treatment course included the insertion of INFUSE Bone Graft followed by 4 to 12 months of bone formation. At 6 months postoperative, mean changes in the bone height from baseline were 7.83 and 9.46 mm for the INFUSE Bone Graft and bone graft groups, respectively. The histology demonstrated that both groups experienced significant formation of new trabecular bone that was biologically and structurally similar to the host site. After 6 months of functional loading, the INFUSE Bone Graft resulted in an implant survival rate of 79%. At 12 months of functional loading, the implant success rates for both groups were comparable with no statistical difference ($P>.05$). Furthermore, no clinically significant adverse events resulted from the use of INFUSE Bone Graft. A large clinical study performed by Fiorellini and colleagues[44] examined the efficacy of 2 doses of rhBMP-2/ACS in 80 patients requiring extraction socket augmentation. rhBMP-2/ACS at 0.75 or 1.5 mg/mL concentrations were examined. The results demonstrated that the 1.5 mg/mL rhBMP-2/ACS treated sites had about 2 times the amount of bone compared with the control group. In addition, histology on core bone biopsies showed no differences between the rhBMP-2–induced bone and native bone. Clinical studies in both maxillary sinus floor augmentations and alveolar ridge augmentation demonstrated that rhBMP-2/ACS at 1.5 mg/mL induced significant bone formation suitable for implant placement. The bone induced by rhBMP-2/ACS was found to be biologically similar to native bone and capable of implant osseointegration and supporting the functional loading of dental prostheses.

MANDIBULAR CONTINUITY RECONSTRUCTION

A 31-year-old man presented with asymptomatic swelling in the right mandible. Radiographic investigation showed a large osteolytic lesion localized in the right mandible (**Figs. 1–3**). A biopsy was taken from the lesion and histologic report revealed it to be an ameloblastoma tumor of the solid multicystic type. The surgical team discussed with the patient all the possible therapeutic options for bone resection and reconstruction. The patient opted for treatment involving growth factor rehabilitation.

Surgical Technique

A full-thickness mucoperiosteal flap was elevated along the defect. The margins of the tumor were both radiographically and clinically identified and the bone was resected 1 cm over the tumor extensions, which totaled nearly 7.5 cm (**Fig. 4**). The anatomic structures were preserved during the resection (**Fig. 5**). Once the underlying ridge was exposed, a mesh was contoured to outline the large defect. It is important to overcorrect by as much as 15% to 20% as some resorption is expected. The underlying ridge is punctured with a small drill to stimulate bleeding. This accomplishes faster integration of the graft as well as supplying additional stem cells to the area. The rhBMP-2 was mixed with the ACS and then modeled on the positioned plate. A portion of the collagen sponge was then cut into small 2- to 3-mm pieces and mixed throughout demineralized bone matrix allograft putty (**Fig. 6**). The rhBMP-2, ACS, and allograft were placed into the mesh and molded according to the patient's mandibular anatomy (**Fig. 7**). No autogenous bone graft was taken from extraoral sites. The mesh and graft material

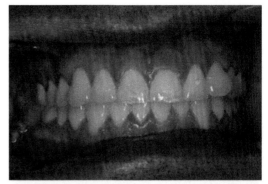

Fig. 2. Clinical examination of the tumor in the vestibular area.

were then secured in place with a minimum of 2 screws. Computed tomography scanning and panographic postoperative radiographs were performed (**Figs. 8** and **9**). The postoperative course was uneventful except for the 1-week postoperative appointment, which revealed edema within the treated area (**Fig. 10**). This sequela is mostly likely explained by the potential of rhBMP-2 to recall inflammatory cells. On examination of the patient at the 3-month follow-up, clinical palpation of the mucosa overlying the resected area revealed a hard indurated surface of the regenerated bone (**Fig. 11**). The patient also exhibited radiographic evidence of bone formation as early as 3 or 4 months postoperatively. Mandibular continuity was regained as demonstrated both clinically and radiographically even at 18 months of follow-up (**Fig. 12**).

MAXILLARY AUGMENTATION

A 49-year-old woman presented for maxillomandibular reconstruction. The patient had a severely atrophic maxilla (**Figs. 13** and **14**) and reported multiple unsuccessful surgeries to increase the vertical dimension. The patient was a smoker

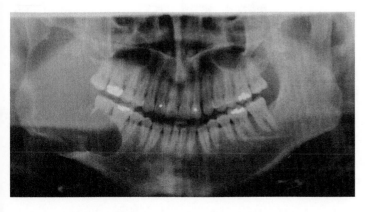

Fig. 1. Preoperative panoramic radiograph investigation shows soft and hard tissue infiltration of lesion in the mandibular area.

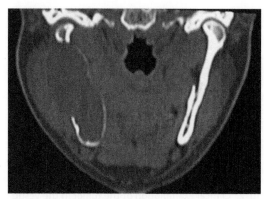

Fig. 3. Computed tomography scan delineates the anatomic extension of the tumor.

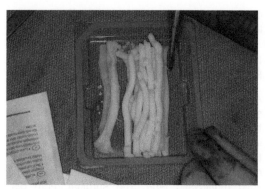

Fig. 6. Recombinant human bone morphogenic protein and carrier preparation.

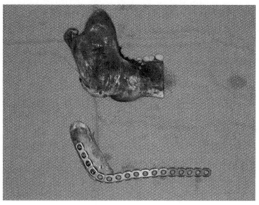

Fig. 4. Ameloblastoma tumor resection showing adequate margins.

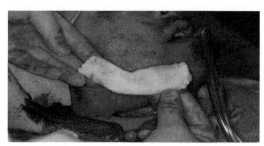

Fig. 7. The biomaterial is modeled conforming to the patient mandibular anatomy.

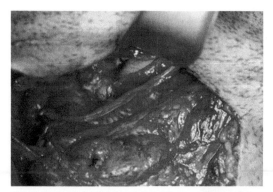

Fig. 5. Anatomic structures have been preserved during surgical resection.

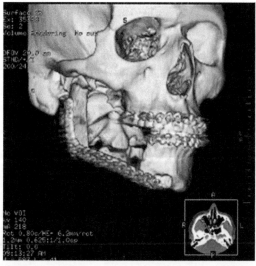

Fig. 8. Computed tomography examination after the plate placement.

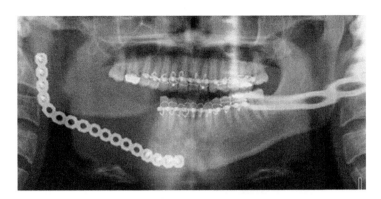

Fig. 9. Panoramic radiograph after defect reconstruction.

and had high expectations. The patient consented for bone augmentation of the maxilla with the addition of allograft and rhBMP-2.

Surgical Technique

A maxillary midcrestal incision was made and the labial flap reflected. A Le Fort I osteotomy was performed to increase the patient's vertical height. The plate and screw positions were modified, maintaining space for future implant placement (**Fig. 15**). Particulate bone allograft was placed in between the bone segments to fill the large resulting defect (**Fig. 16**). No autogenous grafts were harvested. To accelerate healing, an ACS with rhBMP-2 covered the graft (**Fig. 17**). The labial flap was sutured obtaining primary closure.

At the 2-week follow-up, the intraoral clinical examination reveals a better maxillomandibular relationship and improved soft tissue profile (**Figs. 18–20**). Radiographs for implant and prosthetic planning show adequate bone support (**Figs. 21 and 22**). During the implant placement, the labial flap was reflected to reveal stable bone augmentation at the grafted site (**Fig. 23**). The volume reconstructed was enough to consent the placement of 8 dental implants in the maxilla as shown in the postoperative radiograph (**Fig. 24**). It is possible to appreciate the optimal emergence of the prostheses owing to the improved intermaxillary relationship (**Figs. 25 and 26**). The patient was still satisfied at the 5-year follow-up (**Fig. 27**).

CONGENITAL CLEFT CORRECTION

Herford and colleagues[45] described the advantages of the clinical application of rhBMP-2/ACS in a 12-patient study, suggesting that premaxillary osseous clefts can have complete bony repair induced by rhBMP-2. The described technique was used in a case with an 8-year-old boy presenting with a maxillary right cleft alveolar ridge (**Figs. 28 and 29**). The patient's premaxillary cleft was restored with rhBMP-2 in addition to the repair of the oral–nasal fistula. Standard cleft incisions

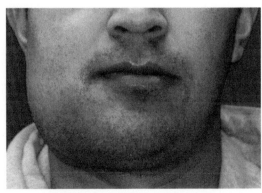

Fig. 10. One-week control revealed significant swelling of the treated area.

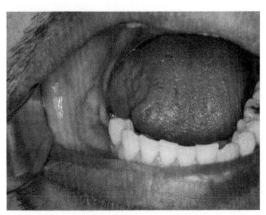

Fig. 11. Clinical follow-up of 18-month control revealed health of the hard and soft tissue.

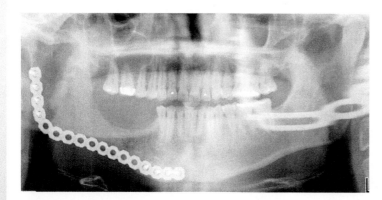

Fig. 12. Radiographic examination 18 months after recombinant human bone morphogenic protein application.

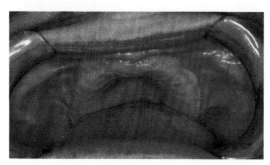

Fig. 13. Clinical examination. Severe atrophy of upper maxilla.

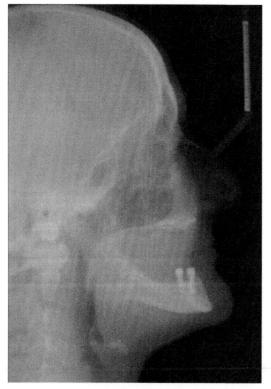

Fig. 14. Lateral cephalometric radiograph showing the high resorption of the maxilla.

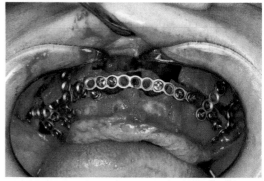

Fig. 15. Intraoperative picture of Le Fort 1 fixation. Plates and screws were positioned for future implant placement.

with labial and palatal incisions were made. Closure of the nasal floor was completed first. BMP with type I collagen sponge was then placed into defects on the facial and palatal defects using a total dose of 4.2 mg of BMP (1.5 mg/mL). Primary closure of mucosal flaps was achieved in order keep the BMP-2 localized and to prevent the compromise of the healing graft.

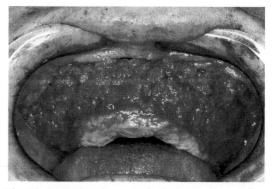

Fig. 16. Particulate bone graft placed over the defect and hardware.

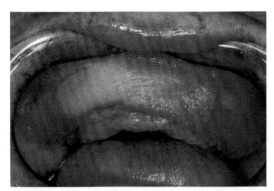

Fig. 17. An absorbable collagen sponge (ASC) with recombinant human bone morphogenic protein.

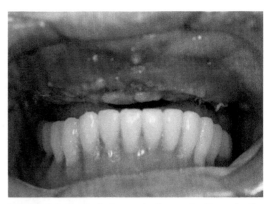

Fig. 20. Intraoral photograph demonstrating a better maxillomandibular relationship.

As in the maxillary reconstruction technique previously described, no autogenous grafts were harvested from the patient, avoiding the need for a donor site and the related morbidity. The cleft was repaired without any particulate allograft, using only the rhBMP-2/ACS to graft the defect (**Figs. 30–32**). The ACS provided a scaffold to maintain the volume necessary to fill the defect. The ACS is compressible in nature and its mechanical support is merely temporary as it resorbs

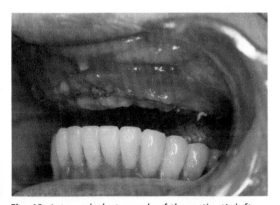

Fig. 18. Intraoral photograph of the patient's left.

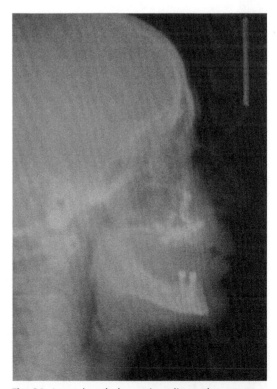

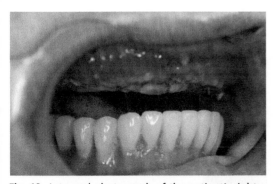

Fig. 19. Intraoral photograph of the patient's right.

Fig. 21. Lateral cephalometric radiograph postoperative showing hardware and a better soft tissue profile.

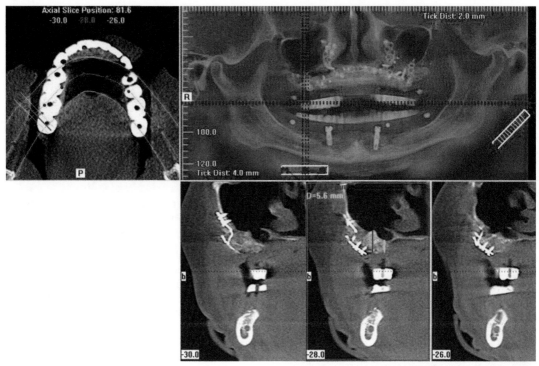

Fig. 22. A computed tomography scan illustrating the stent and resulting implant position, in 3 dimensions.

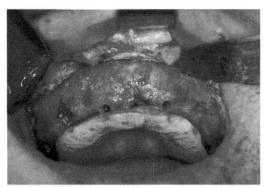

Fig. 23. Soft tissue reflected for implant placement. A vertical and horizontal increase in bone height is appreciable.

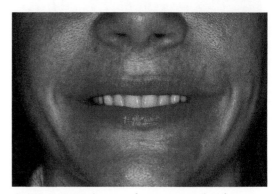

Fig. 25. Extraoral view of patient's smile after prosthetic adaptation.

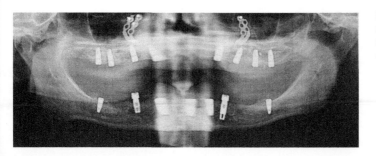

Fig. 24. Panographic radiograph showing 8 implants placed in the maxilla, and 5 in adjunct to the 2 already present in the mandible.

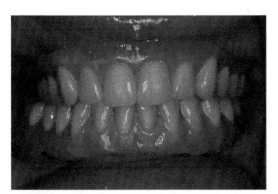

Fig. 26. Intraoral view showing maxillary and mandibular final prostheses.

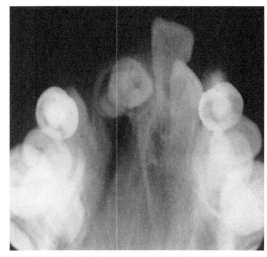

Fig. 29. Occlusal view radiograph of maxillary arch.

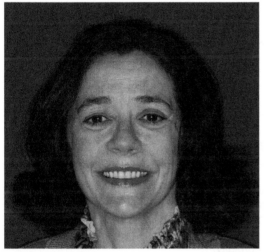

Fig. 27. At 5 years of follow-up. Extraoral view of patient's smile. Lip support is still well-sustained and bony volumes maintained.

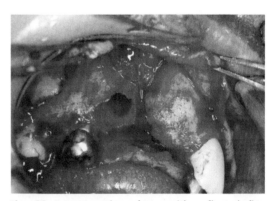

Fig. 30. Intraoperative photo with reflected flap exposing the defect.

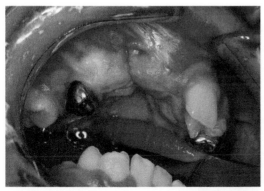

Fig. 28. Preoperative photo of maxillary right cleft.

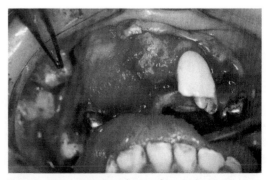

Fig. 31. Intraoperative photo of recombinant human bone morphogenic protein and an absorbable collagen sponge placed into defect.

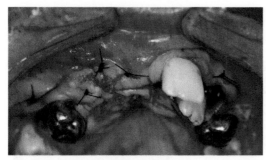

Fig. 32. Intraoperative photograph showing closure of the palatal and labial flaps.

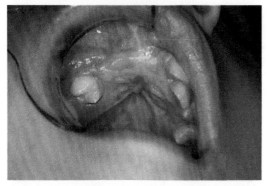

Fig. 33. Postoperative photograph after 6 months demonstrating good healing at the surgical site.

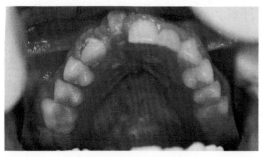

Fig. 34. Intraoral photograph showing an erupting tooth #7 into grafted area at 5 years follow-up.

faster than the formation of bone. However, the bony structure of the cleft is relatively stable compared with a continuity defect or a larger size defect. For this reason, it was possible to use the growth factor associated only with its carrier system without compromising the final clinical result. The graft healed well and supported the eruption of an anterior tooth into the surgical area (**Figs. 33** and **34**). Long-term follow-up of 6 years shows no long-term adverse effects of the BMP (**Fig. 35**). Not all the patients who have been treated with this cleft correction technique underwent orthodontic therapy. The patients treated with rhBMP-2/ACS have very similar radiographs when compared with those treated with iliac crest bone graft.

DISCUSSION

The main advantage of growth factors is not only represented by the avoidance of a donor site, but also by the achievement of better bone healing and quality of bone formation. Use of these factors creates more options in the repair of maxillofacial defects. They can be used to provide increased vascularization, stem cell recruitment, and faster healing at the surgical site. When used in large defects, they reduce the amount of bone needed. The duration of treatment can also be shortened by the application of growth factors. During distraction osteogenesis, treatment is dictated by the rate of bone formation along a vector following latency, distraction, and consolidation. rhBMP-2 has been shown to reduce the time of ossification, shortening treatment time thus reducing patient morbidity.

Documented adverse events related to the use of rhBMP-2 are increased initial facial edema, localized oral erythema, mouth pain, and ecchymosis. The risk of developing a neoplastic lesion could also be considered, and for this reason the application to reconstruct bone defects owing to

Fig. 35. Panoramic radiograph with tooth #7 erupting into grafted site.

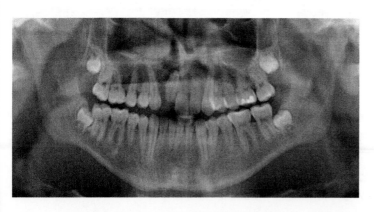

malignant tumor resection should be avoided. Additionally, there are several pathologic processes that probably involve inappropriate VEGF upregulation, such as arteriovascular malformations, tumor growth, and aneurysm formation. Understanding this complex mechanism is the key to developing a tissue-engineered construct that will have appropriate vascular support.

In future applications, the combination of different growth factors will greatly increase the rate of healing. The development of carriers capable of controlling specific release kinetics and patient specific space maintenance will enhance the clinical results, helping to understand the optimal combination and concentration in different cases and defects. The use of growth factors in the treatment of bony defects will continue to be refined owing to their osteoconductive and osteoinducive properties, but for the time being, more studies are necessary to evaluate them fully and provide an evidence-based approach.

SUMMARY

The reconstruction of maxillofacial defects is demanding, because the restoration should meet sound functional and esthetic goals. Biomaterials have been developed to serve as autogenous graft substitutes, while providing a solution that also limits morbidity. Using growth factors extends the reach of allografts or autografts, providing options for large defects and help in maintaining space and permitting earlier calcification. However, more clinical trials are needed to evaluate the long-term effects and the possibility of carcinogenic transformation. The expanding clinical applications of BMPs, the anticipated discovery of new growth factors combined with the better understanding of the biological behavior of important cellular elements, and of pathways of the healing process of tissues would offer novel treatment strategies in the enhancement of tissue regeneration.

REFERENCES

1. Keating JF, Simpson AH, Robinson CM. The management of fractures with bone loss. J Bone Joint Surg Br 2005;87(2):142–50.
2. Taylor GI, Miller GD, Ham FJ. The free vascularized bone graft. A clinical extension of microvascular techniques. Plast Reconstr Surg 1975;55(5):533–44.
3. Rogers GF, Greene AK. Autogenous bone graft: basic science and clinical implications. J Craniofac Surg 2012;23(1):323–7.
4. Roccuzzo M, Ramieri G, Bunino M. Autogenous bone graft alone or associated with titaniummesh for vertical alveolar ridge augmentation: a controlled clinical trial. Clin Oral Impl Res 2007;18:286–94.
5. Wildemann B, Kadow-Romacker A, Pruss A, et al. Quantification of growth factors in allogenic bone grafts extracted with three different methods. Cell Tissue Bank 2007;8(2):107–14.
6. Liu J, Kerns DG. Mechanisms of guided bone regeneration: a review. Open Dent J 2014;8:56.
7. Giannoudis PV, Pountos I. Tissue regeneration. The past, the present and the future. Injury 2005; 36(Suppl 4):S2–5.
8. Giannoudis PV, Einhorn TA, Marsh D. Fracture healing: a harmony of optimal biology and optimal fixation? Injury 2007;38(Suppl 4):S1–2.
9. Giannoudis PV, Tzioupis C. Clinical applications of BMP-7: the UK perspective. Injury 2005; 36(Suppl 3):S47–50.
10. Rutland P, Pulleyn LJ, Reardon W, et al. Identical mutations in the FGFR2 gene cause both Pfeiffer and Crouzon syndrome phenotypes. Nat Genet 1995;9(2):173–6.
11. Harwood PJ, Giannoudis PV. Application of bone morphogenetic proteins in orthopaedic practice: their efficacy and side effects. Expert Opin Drug Saf 2005;4:75–89.
12. Wozney JM. Bone morphogenetic proteins. Prog Growth Factor Res 1989;1:267–80.
13. Coultas L, Chawengsaksophak K, Rossant J. Endothelial cells and VEGF in vascular development. Nature 2005;438:937–45.
14. Street J, Bao M, deGuzman L, et al. Vascular endothelial growth factor stimulates bone repair by promoting angiogenesis and bone turnover. Proc Natl Acad Sci U S A 2002;99:9656–61.
15. Nakagawa M, Kaneda T, Arakawa T, et al. Vascular endothelial growth factor (VEGF) directly enhances osteoclastic bone resorption and survival of mature osteoclasts. FEBS Lett 2000;473:161–4.
16. Barati D, Shariati SRP, Moeinzadeh S, et al. Spatiotemporal release of BMP-2 and VEGF enhances osteogenic and vasculogenic differentiation of human mesenchymal stem cells and endothelial colony-forming cells co-encapsulated in a patterned hydrogel. J Controlled Release 2016;223:126–36.
17. Zhang W, Wang X, Wang S, et al. The use of injectable sonication-induced silk hydrogel for VEGF165 and BMP-2 delivery for elevation of the maxillary sinus floor. Biomaterials 2011; 32(35):9415–24.
18. Du X, Xie Y, Xian CJ, et al. Role of FGFs/FGFRs in skeletal development and bone regeneration. J Cell Physiol 2012;227:3731–43.
19. Nakajima F, Nakajima A, Ogasawara A, et al. Effects of a single percutaneous injection of basic fibroblast growth factor on the healing of a closed femoral shaft fracture in the rat. Calcif Tissue Int 2007;81: 132–8.

20. Kawaguchi H, Oka H, Jingushi S, et al. A local application of recombinant human fibroblast growth factor 2 for tibial shaft fractures: a randomized, placebo-controlled trial. J Bone Miner Res 2012; 25:2735–43.

21. Kaigler D, Avila G, Wisner-Lynch L, et al. Platelet-derived growth factor applications in periodontal and peri-implant bone regeneration. Expert Opin Biol Ther 2011;11:375–85.

22. Tokunaga A, Oya T, Ishii Y, et al. PDGF receptor beta is a potent regulator of mesenchymal stromal cell function. J Bone Miner Res 2008;23:1519–28.

23. Herford AS, Lu M, Akin L, et al. Evaluation of a porcine matrix with and without platelet-derived growth factor for bone graft coverage in pigs. Int J Oral Maxillofacial Implants 2012;27(6):1351–8.

24. Guven G, Gultekin BA, Guven GS, et al. Histologic and Histomorphometric Comparison of Bone Regeneration Between Bone Morphogenetic Protein-2 and Platelet-Derived Growth Factor-BB in Experimental Groups. J Craniofac Surg 2016;27(3): 805–9.

25. Marx RE, Carlson ER, Eichstaedt RM, et al. Platelet-rich plasma: growth factor enhancement for bone grafts. Oral Surg Oral Med Oral Pathol Oral Radiol Endod 1998;85:638–46.

26. Anitua E. The use of plasma-rich growth factors (PRGF) in oral surgery. Pract Proced Aesthet Dent 2001;13:487–93.

27. Del Fabbro M, Bortolin M, Taschieri S, et al. Effect of autologous growth factors in maxillary sinus augmentation: a systematic review. Clin Implant Dent Relat Res 2013;15:205–16.

28. Pocaterra A, Caruso S, Bernardi S, et al. Effectiveness of platelet-rich plasma as an adjunctive material to bone graft: a systematic review and meta-analysis of randomized controlled clinical trials. Int J Oral Maxillofac Surg 2016;45(8):1027–34.

29. Urist MR. Bone: formation by autoinduction. Science 1965;150(3698):893–9.

30. Lavery K, Swain P, Falb D, et al. BMP-2/4 and BMP-6/7 differentially utilize cell surface receptors to induce osteoblastic differentiation of human bone marrow-derived mesenchymal stem cells. J Biol Chem 2008;283(30):20948–58.

31. Kroczek A, Park J, Birkholz T, et al. Effects of osteoinduction on bone regeneration in distraction: results of a pilot study. J Cranio Maxillofacial Surg 2010;38(5):334–44.

32. Friedlaender GE, Perry CR, Cole JD, et al. Osteogenic protein-1 (bone morphogenetic protein-7) in the treatment of tibial nonunions. J Bone Joint Surg Am 2001;83(Suppl 1):S151–8.

33. Govender S, Csimma C, Genant HK, et al. Recombinant human bone morphogenetic protein-2 for treatment of open tibial fractures: a prospective, controlled, randomized study of four hundred and fifty patients. J Bone Joint Surg Am 2002;84: 2123–34.

34. Bourque WT, Gross M, Hall BK. Expression of four growth factors during fracture repair. Int J Dev Biol 1993;37(4):573–9.

35. Boden SD, Zdeblick TA, Sandhu HS, et al. The use of rhBMP-2 in interbody fusion cages: definitive evidence of osteoinduction in humans: a preliminary report. Spine 2000;25(3):376–81.

36. Arosarena OA, Collins WL. Bone regeneration in the rat mandible with bone morphogenetic protein-2: a comparison of two carriers. Otolaryngol Head Neck Surg 2005;132:592–7.

37. Bessa PC, Casal M, Reis RL. Bone morphogenetic proteins in tissue engineering: the road from laboratory to clinic, part II (BMP delivery). J Tissue Eng Regen Med 2008;2:81–96.

38. Barnes B, Boden SD, Louis-Ugbo J. Lower dose of rhBMP-achieves spine fusion when combined with an osteoconductive bulking agent in non-human primates. Spine 2005;30:1127–33.

39. Issa JP, Nascimento C, Bentley MV, et al. Bone repair in rat mandible by rhBMP-2 associated with two carriers. Micron 2008;39:373–9.

40. Herford AS, Stoffella E, Tandon R. Reconstruction of mandibular defects using bone morphogenic protein: can growth factors replace the need for autologous bone grafts? A systematic review of the literature. Plast Surg Int 2011;2011:165824.

41. Tsiridis E, Giannoudis PV. Transcriptomics and proteomics: advancing the understanding of genetic basis of fracture healing. Injury 2006;37(1):S13–9.

42. Boyne PJ, Lilly LC, Marx RE, et al. De novo bone induction by recombinant human bone morphogenetic protein-2 (rhBMP-2) in maxillary sinus floor augmentation. J Oral Maxillofac Surg 2005;63(12): 1693–707.

43. Boyne PJ, Marx RE, Nevins M, et al. A feasibility study evaluating rhBMP-2/absorbable collagen sponge for maxillary sinus floor augmentation. Int J Periodontics Restorative Dent 1997;17(1):11–25.

44. Fiorellini JP, Howell TH, Cochran D, et al. Randomized study evaluating recombinant human bone morphogenetic protein-2 for extraction socket augmentation. J Periodontol 2005;76(4):605–13.

45. Herford AS, Boyne PJ, Rawson R, et al. Bone morphogenetic protein-induced repair of the premaxillary cleft. J Oral Maxillofac Surg 2007;65(11): 2136–41.

Soft Tissue Engineering

Roderick Youngdo Kim, DDS, MD, Sam Seoho Bae, DDS, MD,
Stephen Elliott Feinberg, DDS, MS, PhD*

KEYWORDS

- Soft tissue engineering • Craniomaxillofacial surgery • Oral and maxillofacial surgery
- Head and neck reconstruction • Composite flap • Prelaminated • Lip reconstruction
- Oral mucosa

KEY POINTS

- Barriers that compromise the outcome of soft tissue reconstruction include restoration of vascularity, motor function, sensory innervation, esthetics, and lack of tissue availability.
- Prelamination, prefabrication, and reconstructive innovations such as free tissue transfer have improved the surgical options for patients who sustain avulsion injuries to the craniomaxillofacial structure.
- Complex soft tissue units can be created in vitro and then be implanted onto a muscle bed to create a prelaminated flap in vivo.
- Prelamination/prefabrication of tissue engineered constructs may be the next stage of reconstructive innovation.
- Current proposed methods have the promise of complex tissue reconstruction with volitional, esthetic, and sensate rehabilitation.

INTRODUCTION AND BRIEF HISTORY OF SOFT TISSUE ENGINEERING IN CRANIOMAXILLOFACIAL SURGERY

There is a recognized need to reconstruct and restore complex craniomaxillofacial (CMF) soft tissues that have been damaged and/or disfigured as a consequence of motor vehicle accident, trauma, burn injury, or tumor resection. In trauma, injuries often create extremely complex geometric and avulsion defects, and the anatomic and functional intricacies of CMF composite soft tissue structures such as the lips, eyelids, and nasal complex make the reconstruction particularly challenging for maxillofacial surgeons (**Fig. 1**).

The value of function and esthetics has been a strong factor in driving innovations in CMF surgical techniques and technology. Currently, CMF surgeons frequently use commercially available skin substitutes such as collagen sponges and freeze-dried cadaveric human dermis to replace soft tissue. Unfortunately, these materials do not contain muscle, nerve, or epithelial components and, thus, fail to restore the necessary tissues to allow restoration of the functional properties seen with complex composite soft tissue injuries. Even with advances in both the efficacy and accuracy of surgical techniques and technology such as computed tomography-guided navigation

Disclosure Statement: Drs R.Y. Kim or S.S. Bae, do not have any relevant consultancies, stock ownership or other equity interests, or patent licensing arrangements; Dr S.E. Feinberg is a founding member and chair of the CMF advisory board of Tissue Regeneration Systems. The dermal equivalent used in our studies was obtained gratis from LifeCell Corporation, a subsidiary of Acelity.
Funding: NIH (DE 13417; DE 15784; DE 19431).
Department of Oral & Maxillofacial Surgery, University of Michigan Health System, Towsley Center Rm G1114, 1515 East Medical Center Drive, Ann Arbor, MI 48109-5222, USA
* Corresponding author.
E-mail addresses: sefein@med.umich.edu; sefein@umich.edu

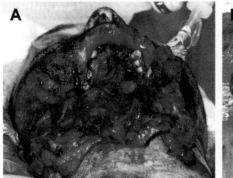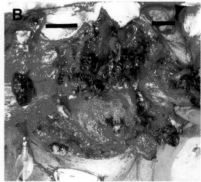

Fig. 1. Complex avulsed defect after self-inflicted gunshot wounds. (*A*) Lower lip only. (*B*) Complete "set" of lips. (*Courtesy of* [*B*] Dr Sean P. Edwards, University of Michigan, Ann Arbor, Michigan.)

systems, 3-dimensional computer-aided surgery, and vascular free tissue transfer, the reconstructive goals of form and function have not been met even in the hands of gifted reconstructive surgeons.[1]

Numerous approaches have been attempted to reconstruct CMF soft tissues, including autogenous, allogeneic, alloplastic, and xenogeneic options.[2] Currently, the majority of soft tissue reconstructive procedures use autologous tissue in the form of tissue grafts and vascularized flaps (pedicle or free), to bring healthy tissue to a compromised defect for optimal healing. However, this has inherent disadvantages of limited tissue availability, color mismatch, and shape incongruity.[3,4]

Several barriers that compromise the outcome of soft tissue reconstruction are the restoration of vascularity, motor function, sensory innervation, esthetics, and the lack of tissue availability. This article focuses on the role that tissue engineering/regenerative medicine (TE/RM) can play in addressing these barriers, and the impediments to optimal tissue reconstruction of complex soft tissue structures. We use the lips as an example to illustrate our points.

CURRENT RECONSTRUCTIVE OPTIONS IN SURGERY

CMF soft tissues form a dynamic complex structure that poses unique challenges in anatomic reconstruction and functional restoration. The lips are an example of a functional soft tissue facial unit that is complex and includes a mucocutaneous junction, innervated muscle, sensory innervation to both skin and mucosa, and blood vessels. Significant loss of lips is both a functional and esthetic concern (**Fig. 2**), because the

neuromuscular control of normal lip structures is required for eating, drinking, talking, and social gesturing.

Avulsion of the lips is a survivable injury. However, without functional lip reconstruction, life for injured individuals is burdened by drooling, food spillage while eating, unintelligible speech, and social rejection. Present lip reconstructions are limited to harvesting existing anatomic units. This includes advancement flaps such as the Karapandzic, rotational flaps such as the Abbe flap, and free vascularized flaps such as the radial forearm fasciocutaneous flap. Functional reconstruction of the lips is so important that when more than 50% of the lips are avulsed or when more than 50% of the transplant team members deem the conventional means of reconstruction impossible or unsatisfactory, face transplantation under lifetime immunosuppression becomes an option.[5]

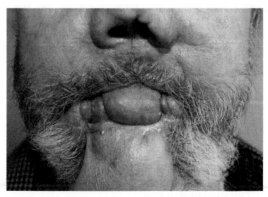

Fig. 2. Reconstructed lips with poor function, complicated by drooling, inability to incise, and unintelligible speech.

The advantages and disadvantages of the contemporary approach to soft tissue reconstruction are:

1. Free grafts (full-thickness skin grafts, split thickness skin grafts, etc):
   a. Pros: Easily harvested, significant tissue availability.
   b. Cons: Poor color match, donor site morbidity, lack of bulk, no function.
2. Local advancement and rotational flaps (Abbe, Karapandzic, Nasolabial, etc):
   a. Pros: Good color match, functional.
   b. Cons: Limited quantity, may require staged surgeries, can lead to microstomia and associated functional deficits in speech and swallowing.
3. Free vascularized tissue transfer (radial forearm, **Fig. 3**):
   a. Pros: excellent vascular pedicle, appropriate tissue thickness, and a method to suspend the lip with the incorporated tendon.
   b. Cons: Long recovery, donor site morbidity, lack of function, poor color match/esthetics, requires specialized surgical skills.
4. Allogeneic tissue transfer/face transplant:
   a. Pros: Good color match, functional tissue, esthetics.
   b. Cons: Requires lifelong immunosuppression, side effects of immunosuppression, long and difficult recovery, donor availability, requires specialized surgical skills and facility.

Currently, the radial forearm free flap with the palmaris longus tendon is a common option for reconstructing total lower lip defects.[6] This becomes inherently difficult in situations where extremities are not available as donor sites, as in battle-wounded soldiers who sustain multiple injuries to both the extremities and CMF structures. The use of the tendon to replace a muscular sphincter is not ideal as it creates a "stiff" lip that lacks the mobility seen in normal lip function.[7] Even in an ideal situation, reconstruction of the lip with a radial forearm lacks the volitional control and offers poor color match.

For large volumes of complex tissue loss, there are limits to the amount of tissue that is transferable. Even after the most extensive free tissue transfer—the total face transfer—function is yet to be ideal. Although total face transplantation may become a tried and true method for restoration of extremely large and complex defects of the head and neck, it requires multiple physical, medical, and psychological therapies and lifetime immunosuppression.[8] Lifetime immunosuppression can result in additional medical comorbidities such as candidiasis, chronic sinusitis, neuropathies, and the development of malignancies.[8,9]

Two closely related but discrete techniques have been used by reconstructive surgeons to address the issue of large and complex composite defects: flap prefabrication and prelamination (**Fig. 4**). Most surgeons have addressed reconstruction of complex soft tissue defects by creating prefabricated flaps with the muscles' own blood supply. In this method, a vascular

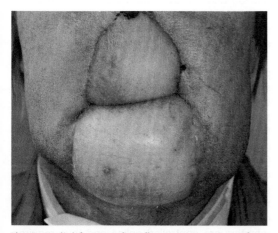

Fig. 3. Radial forearm free flap reconstruction of upper lip avulsion. Lower lip is reconstructed with fibula free flap. (*Courtesy of* Dr Sean P. Edwards, University of Michigan.)

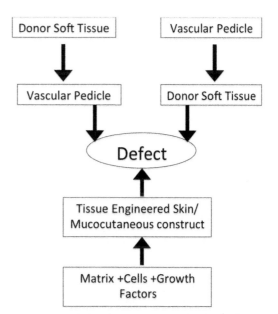

Fig. 4. Prelamination versus prefabrication. (*Adapted from* Garfein ES, Orgill DP, Pribaz JJ. Clinical applications of tissue engineered constructs. Clin Plast Surg 2003;30:485–98.)

carrier is implanted to a new skin territory. Prefabricated flaps have been used in surgery for reconstruction of individual esthetic units such as nose, ear, cheek, lip, and neck.[10–12] With flap prefabrication, a distally ligated vascular pedicle is implanted underneath the desired donor tissue, and after a period of 8 weeks of neovascularization this donor tissue can then be transferred based on the preimplanted vascular pedicle as its axial blood supply.[13]

Prelamination, in contrast, refers to a reconstructive process whereby a 3-dimensional structure is built at a remote donor site by laminating, that is, bonding, different layers of components as composite grafts into a reliable existing axial vascular bed. This does not alter the blood supply to the existing flap.

Flap prefabrication ideally allows the reconstructive surgeon to choose an uninjured donor site with adequate tissue characteristics, an appropriate set of vessels, a motor nerve, as well as a place to fabricate the construct.

Flap prelamination allows reconstruction to begin at a remote donor site, facilitating the structure to mature before transferring the unit en bloc to the defect based on its native axial blood supply. This is important, because the recipient site being reconstructed may lack the blood supply or healthy tissue necessary to support a sophisticated 3-dimensional neoconstruct at the defect site. Furthermore, remote reconstruction in an unscarred vascular bed offers the best chance for the composite grafts to mature.[11] The technique of prelamination is often used in reconstructing structures with multiple functional layers, that is, full-thickness reconstruction of nose, lip, cheek, ear, maxilla, mandible, and trachea.[14]

CURRENT STATE OF SOFT TISSUE ENGINEERING

Major impediments to TE/RM are the limited number of progenitor stem cells that can be obtained from a single donor under current good manufacturing practice (cGMP)-compliant culture systems in a cost-effective way and instituting vascularity and tissue perfusion in a timely manner after implantation. Simply put, the efficiency of producing the base material for assembling the product is lacking.

Engineered human tissue for use in implantation must be manufactured under cGMP standards. cGMP regulations are enforced by the US Food and Drug Administration under Title 21 of the Code of Federal Regulations. Adherence to the cGMP regulations ensures the identity, strength, quality, and purity of cell-based products by requiring that fabrication adequately follows control manufacturing operation standards. cGMPs provide the assurance of proper design, monitoring, and control of manufacturing processes and facilities. This includes establishing strong quality management systems, obtaining appropriate quality raw materials, establishing robust operating procedures, detecting and investigating product quality deviations, and maintaining reliable testing laboratories. This formal system of controls at a laboratory, if adequately put into practice, helps to prevent instances of contamination, mixups, deviations, failures, and errors. This assures that TE/RM products meet their quality standards, and prevents inefficiencies in production (available at: http://www.fda.gov/Drugs/DevelopmentApprovalProcess/Manufacturing/ucm169105.htm). Thus, cGMP is a high standard practice used in laboratories that are based on the regulatory requirements set by the US Food and Drug Administration for the growth and amplification of cells and/or tissues that will be implanted back into humans.

Manufacturing protocols for TE/RM also require detailed and standardized operating procedures of all materials involved in cell growth and tissue fabrication. This process monitors for bacterial and viral contamination, mycoplasma, and requires a certificate of analysis of every chemical that comes into contact with the cells/tissues manufactured in the cGMP facility.

Owing to the limited number of stem cells that can be obtained from a single donor, one of the major challenges on the roadmap for regulatory approval of such medicinal products is the expansion of stem cells using cGMP-compliant culture systems. Manufacturing costs, which include production and quality control procedures, may be the main hurdle for developing cost-effective stem cell therapies for tissue engineered CMF soft tissue constructs.

Currently, bioreactors have gained preference in providing a viable alternative to the traditional static culture systems in that bioreactors provide the required scalability, incorporate monitoring and control tools, and possess the operational flexibility to be adapted to the differing requirements imposed by various clinical applications[15] (**Table 1**). Bioreactor systems are ideal for efficiently producing and amplifying large cell constructs for multiple reasons: compared with a traditional static culture system, bioreactors allow growth beyond the tissue culture flask; culture parameters are controlled online and thus requires less manual upkeep. Furthermore, bioreactors provide the O_2/nutrient exchange, mechanical loading, and cytokine delivery, which allow thicker and more robust tissue constructs. This allows a streamlined and automated production similar to current automotive assembly lines with incorporation of robotic assistance. With the ability to mass produce tissue constructs, TE/RM offers the opportunity to provide effective and unique alternatives to produce custom-made constructs that reestablish and restore function to tissue to or near their preinjured state.

ENGINEERING CRANIOMAXILLOFACIAL SOFT TISSUE: MUCOCUTANEOUS JUNCTION

There are key perceived advantages to reconstructing CMF soft tissue defects using TE/ RM approach:
1. Minimal to no donor site morbidity, because only small pieces of tissue are required to amplify the cells.
2. Faster restoration of function and improvement of outcomes.
   a. Decrease in the number of surgeries needed with a concomitant decrease in operation room time.
   b. Enhancement in the quality, shape, and function of the soft tissue being regenerated.
3. Autochthonous (autogenous) nature of the fabricated soft tissue construct, bypassing the need for immunosuppression.

Currently, TE/RM of human oral mucosa for CMF soft tissue engineering is composed of in vitro fabrication, followed by implantation in vivo. Fabrication of the in vitro mucosa follows the classic triad of soft tissue engineering (**Fig. 5**) that consists of the appropriate cells, scaffold, and physiologically active substances, but now also incorporates the importance of vascularity.[16]

A unique advancement in the reconstruction of lips is predicated on the ability to create a mucocutaneous junction within an autogenous, nonimmunogenic, mucosal/skin tissue equivalent. The ability to fabricate mucosa, skin, and a mucocutaneous human tissue construct has been well documented in the literature.[3] Herein we briefly delineate what is involved in constructing tissue engineered soft tissue equivalents by using a tissue engineered oral mucosa, the ex vivo produced oral mucosa equivalent, as a prototypic example:

- Culture: After harvesting the cells from a 5 mm^2 punch biopsy from the patient, typically from keratinized masticatory mucosa (for lip, from nonkeratinized mucosa), the keratinocytes are isolated, grown, and purified in a defined medium on a decellularized cadaveric human dermis (**Fig. 6**).

- Creation of a mucocutaneous junction: The mucocutaneous junction is created by growing both oral and epidermal keratinocytes on the same piece of dermal equivalent in separate compartments, divided by a physical barrier composed of an inert biocompatible material such as polydimethylsiloxane. Both the oral and skin keratinocytes would be harvested from a punch biopsy in the unattached oral mucosa and retroauricular area, respectively, as a source of keratinocytes. The intermediate area between the skin and keratinocytes is left devoid of cells (**Fig. 7**).
- Growth: The epidermal and oral mucosa keratinocytes are allowed to proliferate and then differentiate (stratify) by altering the concentration of calcium in the medium.
- On removal of the polydimethylsiloxane barrier, the oral and skin keratinocytes are allowed to comingle in the unseeded, acellular, area and form a third distinct regional site, a vermillion.
- These 3 phenotypically distinct anatomic sites, skin, vermillion, and oral mucosa form a mucocutaneous junction that can be used in flap prelamination in preparation for lip reconstruction (**Fig. 8**).

These tissue engineered constructs promise the potential for regeneration and reconstruction of simple as well as complex tissues or organs, using cells and/or growth factors implanted into or onto suitable carrier scaffolds.[3]

A FUTURISTIC APPROACH TO CONSTRUCTION OF CRANIOMAXILLOFACIAL SOFT TISSUE COMPOSITES USING A TISSUE ENGINEERING/REGENERATIVE MEDICINE APPROACH

Along with the advancement of surgical innovations of prefabrication and prelamination, TE/RM advances are now becoming intertwined to create "designer" flaps. Our proposed methodology to functional lip reconstruction would consist of the following:

1. After subject recruitment, we will take two 1.0 cm circular punch biopsies: the posterior auricular area for autogenous skin keratinocytes and the buccal (cheek) mucosa for autogenous oral keratinocytes.
2. Fabrication of a mucocutaneous (M/C) construct, in vitro, in a cGMP facility with autogenous skin and oral keratinocytes using standard operating procedures and an appropriate template for M/C fabrication that would

Table 1
Engineering parameters in bioreactor's design: a critical aspect in tissue engineering

Bioreactor Type	General Descriptions	Mass Transfer Mechanism	Shear Stress	Special Usage	Tissue	Considerations
Static culture	Batch culture with no flow of nutrient	Diffusion (high)	Very low	Cell proliferation		Homogeneous structure of cell constructs and nutrient diffusion limitations
Stirred flasks	Magnetically stirring of medium	Convection (high)	High	Dynamic seeding of scaffolds	Cartilage	Appropriate scaffold and balance between increasing mass transfer and modulating shear stresses

Rotating wall		Rotating at a speed so the constructs in the reactor are maintained "stationary" in a state of continuous free fall	Convection (high)	Low	Tissue constructs which need dynamic laminar flow	Cartilage, bone and skin	Operating conditions (e.g., speed of rotating) especially for growing large tissue mass
Perfusion		Flow of medium over or through a cell population or bed of cells	Convection (moderate) and diffusion (high)	Moderate	Tissues physicochemically and environmentally relevant to human tissues	Epithelial cells, intestinal, bone, cartilage, and arteries	Seeding and attachment of human cells especially within the scaffold body

(From Salehi-Nik N, Amoabediny G, Pouran B, et al. Engineering parameters in bioreactor's design: a critical aspect in tissue engineering. Biomed Res Int 2013;2013:762132.)

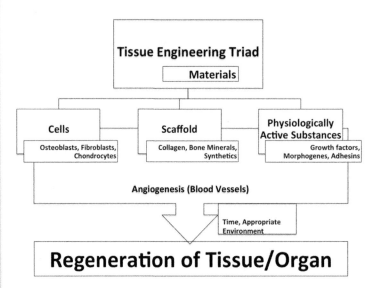

Fig. 5. Tissue engineering triad.

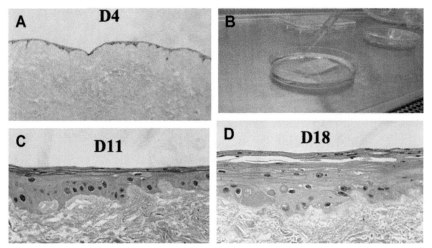

Fig. 6. Culturing of ex vivo produced oral mucosa equivalent (EVPOME) after seeding of oral keratinocytes onto acellular dermal matrix. (*A*) Four days submerged in culture after seeding of oral keratinocytes (Day 4). (*B*) EV-POME raised to an air–liquid interface. (*C*) EVPOME grown at an air–liquid interface for 7 days (day 11). (*D*) EV-POME grown for additional 7 days (day 18) showing increased cell stratification.

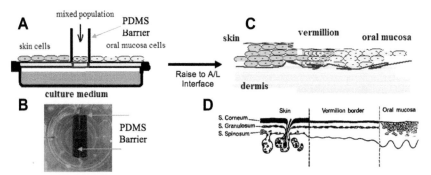

Fig. 7. (*A*) Two-dimensional (2D) culture. (*B*) View from the top of the 2D culture. (*C*) Schematic of *A*, when it is raised to an air–liquid (A/L) interface to become a 3-dimensional organotypic construct. (*D*) A diagrammatic representation of histology of a full thickness lip. ([*C*] *From* Binnie WH, Lehner T. Histology of the muco-cutaneous junction at the corner of the human mouth. Arch Oral Biol 1970;15:777–86; with permission.)

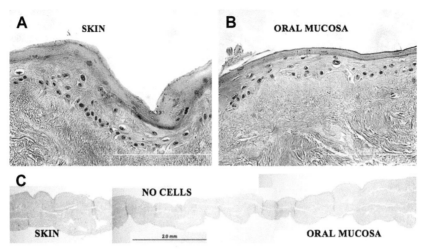

Fig. 8. Note differences in keratinization patterns between (*A*) skin and (*B*) oral mucosa when grown under the same culture conditions on the same dermal construct (*C*). In (*C*) we can see the acellular area that will eventually form the vermillion after the skin and oral cell populations migrate towards one another.

address the size and geometry of the defect to be reconstructed (**Fig. 9**).

3. Grafting of the ex vivo fabricated M/C construct onto the latissimus dorsi muscle (LDM), as a laminate, to create an innervated prevascularized prefabricated (IPP) flap. The implantation of the M/C construct will be placed parallel to the muscle fibers of the LDM as well as parallel to the motor nerve and blood supply based on the thoracodorsal vessels and motor nerve. The parallel position of the neurovascular bundle and M/C construct will facilitate the surgical

Fig. 9. Template for making a complete "set" of lips.

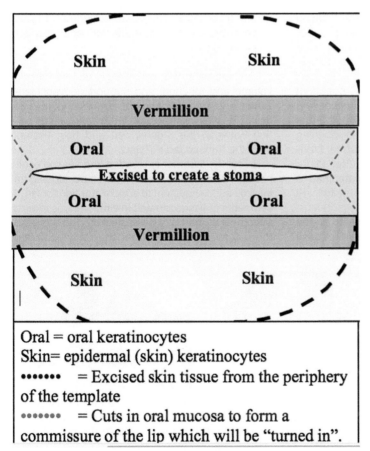

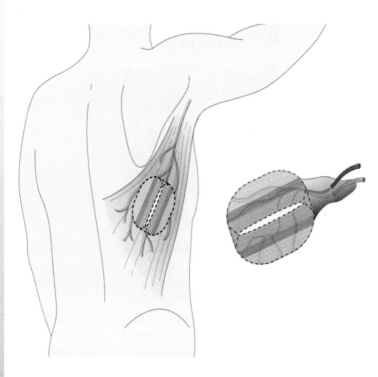

Fig. 10. Lamination to the latissimus dorsi, paralleling the muscle fibers and along the thoracodorsal neurovascular bundle. (*From* Kim RY, Fasi AC, Feinberg SE. Soft tissue engineering in craniomaxillofacial surgery. Ann Maxillofac Surg 2014;4:4–8; with permission.)

inset of the flap and the functional dilation and contraction of the muscle fibers. The location of the M/C construct is planned to be just below the angle of the scapula/scapula tip, to allow for an appropriate length of the neurovascular pedicle (**Fig. 10**).

4. Creation of a stoma within the M/C construct and LDM such that the long axis of the opening is parallel to the muscle fibers to simulate the orbicularis oris muscle. The stoma or opening will be maintained with a silastic obturator fabricated from a 3-dimensional printer (**Fig. 11**).
5. Harvesting of the designer prelaminated flap at 2 to 3 weeks after implantation, per preliminary animal data.
6. Perform a microvascular free transfer to the recipient site containing the thoracodorsal artery, vein and motor nerve to the external carotid or facial artery, external jugular or facial vein, and a branch of the facial nerve, respectively (**Fig. 12**).

This approach will successfully restore muscle volume and function, and support neovascularization and reinnervation of regenerated muscle tissue, as well as structural and functional integration between the regenerated and host tissues from the transposed IPP flap.

Presently, a barrier in creating large tissue engineered constructs is the difficulty in developing an in vivo vascular system to supply nutrition for large segments of tissue created in vitro. Various in vitro culture systems have been designed to simulate the natural environment, but they only allow the

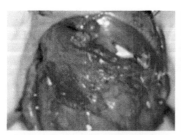
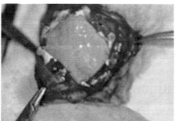
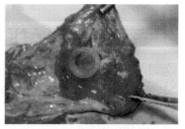

Fig. 11. (*Left*) Intact latissimus dorsi muscle on an athymic rat that will be the recipient bed for the laminate. (*Middle*) Graft of the dermal equivalent onto the latissimus dorsi muscle showing the opaqueness indicative of lack of vascularity. (*Right*) Three weeks after implantation showing increase vascularity to the dermal graft and placement of an obturator to create a stoma.

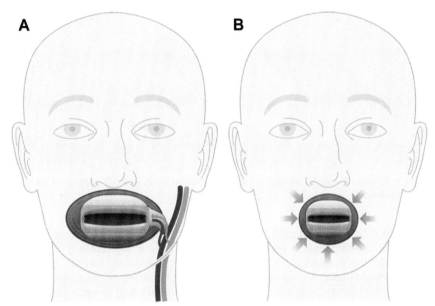

Fig. 12. (*A*) Anastomosis of thoracodorsal artery with a branch of external carotid artery and internal jugular vein. The motor nerve is anastomosed to the facial nerve (not shown). (*B*) Muscle contraction to simulate orbicularis oris function on stimulation of the latissimus dorsi muscle thoracodorsal nerve.

growth of small, uncomplicated pieces of tissue. Vascularization and nutrition are significant issues, limiting the size and complexity of tissue engineered constructs that can be successfully transplanted after it is grown in vitro.[17] Ex vivo fabrication of composite soft tissue thicker than a few millimeters are vulnerable because diffusion and imbibition are not effective means of supplying the central parts of the neotissue.

The IPP approach addresses a major impediment to the successful tissue engineering of complex composite soft tissue grafts: "adequate tissue perfusion," that is, the vascular supply, through prefabrication and prelamination. The use of microvascular free transfer of prelaminated/prefabricated "designer flaps" creates instant perfusion of the transposed tissue once the anastomosis is complete.

By placing the laminate composed of the mucocutaneous construct on the LDM, subcutaneously onto the muscle bed, we are using the body as an in situ bioreactor to address the issue of vascularity and tissue perfusion by allowing ingrowth of vessels to develop a microcapillary system into the laminate that is, based on the major vessels, artery and vein, of the LDM, the thoracodorsal artery. Several studies show the efficacy for the placement of either strips of buccal mucosa[18–20] or tissue engineered oral mucosa in the successful creation of radial forearm prelaminated flaps.[21] Tark and colleagues[22] showed that it was possible to create a prefabricated skin flap using an

acellular dermal matrix in conjunction with cultured keratinocytes as we propose in this article. Tark and associates also noted a vascularization period of 2 weeks with evidence of fibroblast infiltration and the presence of luminal spaces surrounded by capillary endothelium characteristic of neovascularization of the matrix. This is similar to what we noted in our own SCID mouse study.[23] Furthermore, in our IPP rat model we see that the underlying muscle integrates completely with the overlying dermal equivalent (**Fig. 13**), and should as well with the cellular 3-dimensional mucocutaneous constructs in humans (unpublished data).

DEVELOPMENT OF DEVICES TO ASSESS TISSUE PERFUSION FOR SUBCUTANEOUSLY PLACED, BURIED FLAPS

A disadvantage of "burying" the designer flap underneath the skin is that maturation occurs in a position that is not readily observable. There are few options of clinical assessment to evaluate flap maturation that exist, including Doppler examination or surgical exploration, which has inherent morbidity and repeated anesthesia, as well as disturbance of the surgical bed. There are developments of devices such as Raman and diffuse reflectance spectroscopy that may allow for noninvasive measure of graft viability/perfusion through the native skin.[24–26] These probes mimic pen Doppler devices in size, and via a transcutaneous approach, are able to detect the vascular flow and

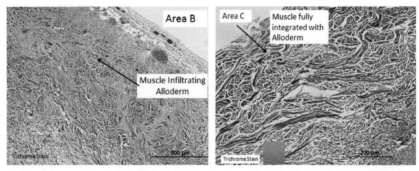

Fig. 13. Histologic evidence of muscle infiltration into the dermal equivalent. (*Courtesy of* Melanie Urbanchek, PhD, University of Michigan.)

the reflectance created by red blood cells. These Doppler monitors use specific laser wavelengths that penetrate through the overlying skin and to the maturing prelaminated tissue. The device captures the reflectance wavelength, which is derived from the concentration of oxyhemoglobin and deoxyhemoglobin. Other monitors detect the high-frequency fluctuations through the movement of red blood cells through the vascular channels (laser speckle), confirming vascular flow (**Fig. 14**).

SECONDARY CHALLENGES IN FUNCTIONAL TISSUE ENGINEERED CRANIOMAXILLOFACIAL SOFT TISSUE

By burying the flap and allowing inosculation, imbibition, and ultimately prefabrication of the prelaminated tissue engineered constructs on the LDM to occur, we create a composite soft tissue graft of epithelium, dermis, and muscle. By harvesting the thoracodorsal motor nerve with the artery and vein, and anastomosing the motor nerve to the facial nerve, we address another barrier to creation of functional lips, that is, the motor function.

From preliminary animal data we have serendipitously noted that there is evidence of sensory nerve ingrowth into the soft tissue composite graft following the microvascular capillary network. This would be consistent with Siemionow and colleagues,[27] who showed that nearly normal sensory recovery can be expected following facial allotransplantation with or without repair of the sensory nerves. We, thus, expect a similar scenario to occur in the autogenous IPP flaps (**Fig. 15**).

Fig. 14. Diagrammatic representation of ex vivo produced oral mucosa equivalent monitored transcutaneously with laser probes.

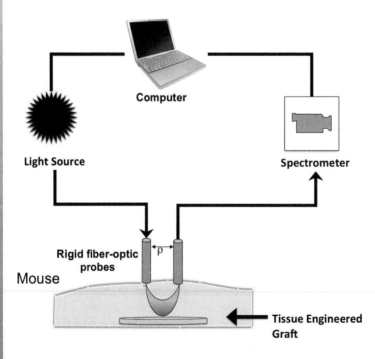

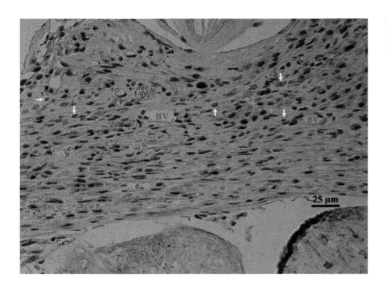

Fig. 15. Sensory nerve ingrowth. BV, blood vessel; yellow arrow, sensory nerve.

Last, in terms of color match, although the initially grafted mucocutaneous equivalent is quite pale compared with native tissue, after revascularization has occurred after grafting, the dermal equivalent gains marked color change. In our previous studies with ex vivo produced oral mucosa equivalent grafts, the ex vivo produced oral mucosa equivalent conferred more esthetically pleasing gingival graft in both hue (color) and thickness when compared with the conventional autologous palatal free gingival graft.[28] Therefore, we expect the tissue engineered IPP flap to also obtain comparable esthetic results (**Fig. 16**).

LIMITATIONS

As with any innovation, there are many hurdles that remain to be addressed and challenges to overcome. The main issues present include the interplay between the timing, regional applicability/dissemination, and regulation.

For timing, in general it takes about 28 days from the harvest of cell to implantation. Because we are using patient-specific cells (autogenous), this requires amplification of cells before prefabrication and prelamination. We need a device that can automatically, consistently, and economically produce cells that have the maximum viability and uniformity for use in TE/RM; cGMP based on bioreactors may be the solution. However, establishing the reliability of mass production, and the fact that current technologies of evaluation techniques for cell viability has not been challenged, we require further data from currently proposed clinical trials.

Second, the technology to develop and fabricate tissue engineered devices from stem cells and progenitor cells originated from academic research centers and small startup companies. A main barrier to TE/RM devices to date is the cost for their fabrication, which is due to the restrictive specifications of culture condition, poor streamlined production process, and high facility maintenance cost.[15] Currently, the "designer" free flaps are a time consuming, multidisciplinary, and specialized endeavor. It may be sustained only in large institutions, because it requires coordination

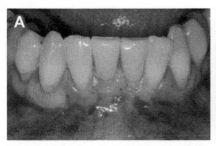
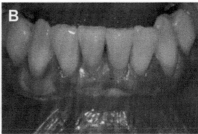

Fig. 16. (*A*) Photographs before and (*B*) after surgery (6 weeks) of grafted ex vivo produced oral mucosa equivalent (EVPOME). Note color rendition. (*Adapted from* Izumi K, Neiva R, Feinberg SE. Intraoral grafting of a tissue engineered human oral mucosa. Int J Oral Maxillofac Implants 2013;28(5):e295–303.)

between the specialized "bench" team with the surgical team.

Another impediment to acceptance is that it takes an additional 2 to 3 weeks for prelaminated flaps to become neovascularized to be transferred en bloc with the native flap with its own blood supply. This is a relatively lengthy amount of time and, in certain situations, the patient will not or cannot wait until the tissue is ready to be transplanted. There are multiple instances where the duration of fabrication and prelamination of the tissue engineered flap would be an issue, such as seen in reconstruction of ablative defects from malignancy. There are data that show that, after 6 weeks from diagnosis, the prognosis worsens if no treatment is rendered.[29,30] Thus, an immediate reconstruction with a tissue engineered graft is currently impractical.

Last, the absolute requirement of using cGMP manufacturing protocol consistent with US Food and Drug Administration regulatory guidelines and complex commercialization strategies make most of these "living composite (combinational) products" similar to an orphan drug and there is little or no financial incentive for a company to participate in their commercialization. Thus, it is necessary to coordinate the bringing of this type of TE/RM product to market developed by researchers, in partnership with the government (Department of Defense). These partnerships will need to reside in tertiary regional clinical centers in the United States that have a major university and a Veteran's Administration Hospital in close proximity. These TE/RM centers will need to have a functional cGMP (clean room) facility on site. The cGMP facility will fabricate the in vitro M/C constructs for implantation for the development of IPP flaps. This approach will create an administrative and physical infrastructure for dissemination of this novel technology to the military and the public in a cost-effective and efficient manner. The designated TE/RM surgical centers will be regional referral facilities that contain the necessary manufacturing (cGMP) facilities to fabricate the combinational devices and have the surgical expertise for use in restoration of lost tissue and function seen in wounded warriors and civilians in need of this unique and novel technology.

We believe our unique approach to the fabrication of composite soft tissue grafts addresses the issues of complexity, functionality, and vascularity, which have prevented TE/RM from entering the clinical arena thus far.

FUTURE OUTLOOK

Through our current experience and available literature, we are 1 step closer to achieving a true bench-to-bedside engineered soft tissue that would address defects from congenital, ablative, and avulsed injuries. In the head and neck region, the most exciting current endeavors include "designer" free flaps such as the prefabricated/prelaminated flaps, which would allow reconstructions of complex composite defects consisting of bone, muscle, fascia, and mucosa or skin. This also has the promise of a sensate flap.

With prefabricated, prelaminated flaps demonstrating great success in complex CMF soft tissue

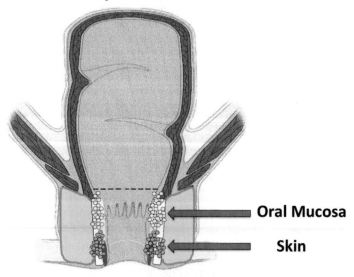

Neo Sphincter after Lamination

→ **Oral Mucosa**

→ **Skin**

Fig. 17. Schematic design of a neoanus. The latissimus dorsi muscle is rolled up to create the lumen. (*Courtesy of* Melanie Urbanchek, PhD, University of Michigan.)

reconstruction in the future, further studies based on histologic analysis of neurovascular ingrowth and development will yield protocols for the next generation of reconstructive surgery. This would develop a platform of technology for soft tissue reconstruction. Our proposed new technologies involving the next generation of bioreactors, optical technologies, and economical production of tissue equivalents, will yield a product for clinical use in TE/RM for military and commercialization. In addition, these novel techniques can be applicable beyond the CMF region.

One of the natural derivations from the study of lips is that there are various sphincters and mucocutaneous junctions in the body. During our study with the Department of Defense, we became well aware of devastating perineal wounds suffered by our warriors in combat. These defects are incredibly difficult to reconstruct, and include straight closure of the perineum and colostomy, or reconstruction with gracilis myocutaneous rotational flap, which are prone to wound breakdown and persistent infection.[31] Furthermore, even with reconstruction of the skin and obturation of the dead space, many of these soldiers lack sphincter control, and suffer incontinence (**Fig. 17**).

Using techniques and mistakes learned from the creation of lips, we have expanded our work in a multidisciplinary team to develop tissue constructs composed of muscle, anal mucosa, and neural tissue to fabricate an anal tissue equivalent for reconstruction of the pelvic floor. We have been involved in the Armed Forces Institute of Regenerative Medicine (AFIRM II) to address these defects, highlighting the applicability of the knowledge gained from maxillofacial tissue engineering and reconstruction to other areas of the body, that is, eyelids and the vagina.

SUMMARY

There is a continued need for reconstruction of complex soft tissue defects of the head and neck tissue. There have been advances in reconstruction through regenerative medicine, tissue engineering, and advanced surgical reconstruction. However, each of these endeavors has its positive and negative aspects. Throughout our past and present studies, the issue of immunosuppression and graft rejection has been addressed by harvesting the patient's own cells. We have also addressed the junctions involved in mucocutaneous transition, by creating a tissue engineered mucocutaneous junction. We have addressed vascularity of engineered tissue by the prefabrication and prelamination and transfer via free tissue transfer. We are also creating sensate and

volitional tissue by prelamination, microneuroanastomsis, and studying the ingrowth of sensory nerves, which should follow the developing microcapillary system.

However, many hurdles remain. Further studies are needed to address function and sensation as well as robust phase II and III multicenter clinical trials to evaluate the viability and effectiveness of development of regional centers to disseminate this type of specialized therapy. In addition, long-term studies are needed to assess color, function, and durability of patients with prelaminated/prefabricated rotational and free flaps.

Although still in its infancy for clinical application, the promise of complex tissue reconstruction, sensate and functional tissue, and ultimately esthetically pleasing engineered tissue is a worthwhile endeavor that we continue to pursue.

REFERENCES

1. Rodriguez ED, Bluebond-Langner R, Park JE, et al. Preservation of contour in periorbital and midfacial craniofacial microsurgery: reconstruction of the soft-tissue elements and skeletal buttresses. Plast Reconstr Surg 2008;121(5):1738–47 [discussion: 1748–9].

2. Bagheri S, Bell B, Khan H. Current therapy in oral and maxillofacial surgery. ch 9. In: Tissue engineering. St Louis (MO): Elsevier Saunders; 2011. p. 79–91. ISBN: 978-1-4160-2527-6.

3. Izumi K, Song J, Feinberg SE. Development of a tissue-engineered human oral mucosa: from the bench to the bedside. Cells Tissues Organs 2004; 176:134–52.

4. Balasundarama I, Al-Hadad I, Parmar S. Recent advances in reconstructive oral and maxillofacial surgery. Br J Oral Maxillofac Surg 2012;50(8):695–705.

5. Wo L, Bueno E, Pomahac B. Facial transplantation: worth the risks? A look at evolution of indications over the last decade. Curr Opin Organ Transpl 2015;20(6):615–20.

6. Faria JC, Scopel GP, Alonso N, et al. Muscle transplants for facial reanimation: rationale and results of insertion technique using the palmaris longus tendon. Ann Plast Surg 2009;63:148–52.

7. Trussler AP, Kawamoto HK, Wasson KL, et al. Upper lip augmentation: palmaris longus tendon as an autologous filler. Plast Reconstr Surg 2008;121(3): 1024–32.

8. Garrett GL, Beegun I, D'Souza A. Facial transplantation: historical developments and future directions. J Laryngol Otol 2015;129:206–11.

9. Kim TB, Pletcher SD, Goldberg AN. Head and neck manifestations in the immunocompromised host. In: Flint PW, Haughey BH, Lund VJ, et al, editors. Cummings otolaryngology: head and neck surgery.

5th edition. Philadelphia: Mosby/Elsevier; 2010. p. 209–29 (225–226).

10. Teot L, Cherenfant E, Otman S, et al. Prefabricated vascularized supraclavicular flaps for face resurfacing after postburns scarring. Lancet 2000;355: 1695–6.

11. Pribaz JJ, Fine N, Orgill DP. Flap prefabrication in the head and neck: a 10-year experience. Plast Reconstr Surg 1999;103:808–20.

12. Evans DM. Facial reconstruction after a burn injury using two circumferential radial forearm flaps, and a dorsalis pedis flap for the nose. Br J Plast Surg 1995;48:471–6.

13. Guo L, Pribaz JJ. Clinical flap prefabrication. Plast Reconstr Surg 2009;124:e340–50.

14. Vranckx JJ, Delaere P, Vanderpoorten V. Prefabrication and prelamination procedures for larynx and tracheal reconstruction. Paper presented at: Fourth Congress of the World Society for Reconstructive Microsurgery. Buenos Aires, Argentina, October 23–25, 2005.

15. dos Santos FF, Andrade PZ, da Silva CL, et al. Bioreactor design for clinical-grade expansion of stem cells. Biotechnol J 2013;8(6):644–54.

16. Payne KF, Balasundaram I, Deb S, et al. Tissue engineering technology and its possible applications in oral and maxillofacial surgery. Br J Oral Maxillofac Surg 2014;52(1):7–15.

17. Spector M. Basic principles of tissue engineering. Chapter 1: tissue engineering. Chicago: Quintessence Publishing Co., Inc; 1999.

18. Millesi W, Rath T, Millesi-Schobel G, et al. Reconstruction of the floor of the mouth with a fascial radial forearm flap, prelaminated with autologous mucosa. Int J Oral Maxillofac Surg 1998;27:106.

19. Rath T, Millesi W, Millesi-Schobel G, et al. Mucosal prelaminated flaps for physiological reconstruction of intraoral defects after tumour resection. Br J Plast Surg 1997;50:303.

20. Rath T, Millesi W, Millesi-Schobel G, et al. Mucosal prelamination of a radial forearm flap for intraoral reconstruction. J Reconstr Microsurg 1997;13:507.

21. Lauer G, Schimming R, Gellrich N-C, et al. Prelaminating the fascial radial forearm flap by using tissue-engineered mucosa: improvement of donor and recipient sites. Plast Reconstr Surg 2001;108:1564.

22. Tark KC, Chung S, Shin KS, et al. Skin flap prefabrication using acellular dermal matrix and cultured keratinocytes in a porcine model. Ann Plast Surg 2000;44:392–7.

23. Izumi K, Feinberg SE, Teraski H, et al. Evaluation of transplanted tissue-engineered oral mucosa equivalents to SCID mice. Tissue Eng 2003;9:161–72.

24. Khmaladze A, Ganguly A, Kuo S, et al. Tissue-engineered constructs of human oral mucosa examined by Raman spectroscopy. Tissue Eng Part C Methods 2013;19:299–306.

25. Khmaladze A, Kuo S, Kim RY, et al. Human oral mucosa tissue-engineered constructs monitored by Raman fiber-optic probe. Tissue Eng Part C Methods 2015;21(1):46–51.

26. Karthik V, Gurjar R, Kuo S, et al. Sensing vascularization of ex-vivo produced oral mucosal equivalent (EVPOME) skin grafts in nude mice using optical spectroscopy. Proc. SPIE 8926, Photonic Therapeutics and Diagnostics X, 89260I, March 4, 2014.

27. Siemionow M, Gharb BB, Rampazzo A. Pathways of sensory recovery after face transplantation. Plast Reconstr Surg 2011;127(5):1875–89.

28. Izumi K, Neiva R, Feinberg SE. Intraoral grafting of a tissue engineered human oral mucosa. Int J Oral Maxillofac Implants 2013;28(5):e295–303.

29. Ang KK, Trotti A, Brown BW, et al. Randomized trial addressing risk features and time factors of surgery plus radiotherapy in advanced head-and-neck cancer. Int J Radiat Oncol Biol Phys 2001; 51(3):571–8.

30. Peters LJ, Withers HR. Applying radiobiological principles to combined modality treatment of head and neck cancer–the time factor. Int J Radiat Oncol Biol Phys 1997;39(4):831–6.

31. Wong DS. Reconstruction of the perineum. Ann Plast Surg 2014;73(Suppl 1):S74–81.

New Frontiers in Biomaterials

R. Gilbert Triplett, DDS, PhD[a,b,]*, Oksana Budinskaya, DDS[c]

KEYWORDS

- Tissue engineering • Regenerative medicine • Biomaterials • Angiogenesis
- Nanophase biomaterial • Atmospheric cold plasma

KEY POINTS

- Tissue loss due to trauma or pathology or for congenital purposes necessitates the replacement of form and function, and this has led to the development of tissue engineering and regenerative medicine.
- Grafting materials and techniques have undergone a rapid evolution from simply replacing tissues to stimulating a response from the host.
- These developments are promising in that previously unattainable results in skin, nerve, muscle, and specialized tissue bioengineering are within reach.

INTRODUCTION

A biomaterial in medical terminology is "any natural or synthetic material (which includes polymer or metal) that is intended for introduction into living tissues as part of a medical device or implant" (for example artificial heart or temporomandibular joint). Biomaterials from a health care perspective can be defined as "materials that possess some novel properties that makes them appropriate to come into immediate contact with the living tissue without eliciting an adverse immune rejection reaction."[1]

Tissue loss in the craniomaxillofacial region occurs frequently from disease, trauma, and congenital abnormalities. This loss induces serious physiologic and psychological consequences for patients and their families.[2] Reconstruction of this area to an esthetic and functional state is the goal of the reconstructive surgeon.

Historically, tissue replacement with biomaterials in the craniomaxillofacial region focused on the physical properties of the material itself, such as inertness, malleability, and strength. Over the past 35 years, both the science and funding of biomaterials have seen incredible growth. Biomaterial science has evolved through the research, clinical experience, and collaboration between researchers and surgeons. Recently research has redirected its focus on the biologic interactions of implant materials with the surrounding tissue and cells.[3]

In the past, removable or implanted prostheses used to obturate and replace tissues in this region were fabricated with metals and ceramics. Although they provided an improved esthetic and functional state, they had their limitations. These materials were believed "inert" and, therefore, incapable of eliciting an unfavorable reaction from the host tissue. It is now recognized that various "inert" materials can change physically and chemically after implantation and, from a biological perspective, no material should be considered truly inert.[4]

Disclosure Statement: The authors have nothing to disclose.
^a Department of Oral and Maxillofacial Surgery, Texas A&M – College of Dentistry, 3302 Gaston Avenue, Dallas, Texas 75246, USA; ^b Department of Surgery, Division of Dentistry, Baylor University Medical Center, Dallas, Texas, USA; ^c Department of Diagnostic Sciences, Baylor College of Dentistry, 3302 Gaston Avenue, Room 215, Dallas, TX 75246, USA
* Corresponding author.
E-mail address: Gtriplett@bcd.tamhsc.edu

Numerous advances have been made in the area of biomaterials and tissue engineering; however, the complexity of human tissues and organs has not been simple to unscramble and mechanisms and interaction between the tissues, cells, and various factors are still being discovered. This article discusses the exciting and novel areas of discovery, first discussing the basic concepts of biomaterials, their development, and their potential implementation to understand the endless possibilities in this field with their current limitations and shortcomings.

BACKGROUND

The first generation of biomaterials evolved during the 1960s and 1970s and initially served mainly as medical implants. Basic goals during the fabrication of these biomaterials consisted in maintaining a balance between physical and mechanical properties with minimal toxicity to host tissues.[5] Ideal properties of the first-generation biomaterials were (1) appropriate mechanical properties, (2) resistance to corrosion in an aqueous environment, and (3) not eliciting toxicity or carcinogenicity in living tissue. Second-generation biomaterials were developed to also be bioactive. Substantial progress was observed in the application for orthopedic and dental use. Examples include bioactive glasses, ceramics, polymers, glass-ceramics, and composites.[1,5]

Current developments with biomaterial technology are now translating into the expansion of a third-generation of biomaterials that can stimulate a specific cellular response.[1] This research is focused on the development and improvement of scaffolding, the delivery of site-specific cells, and the use of necessary growth factors and various molecules to an area needing regeneration. These scaffolds are used as extracellular matrixes (ECMs) to provide 3-D supporting structure to the cells, resulting in a "tissue construct." Various biomaterial scaffolds are being investigated and include naturally occurring biodegradable polymers, synthetic organic biodegradable polymers, hydrogels, and synthetic bioactive glass and ceramics.

These biomaterial scaffolds have been demonstrated to have an effect on the cellular activity of cells within and adjacent to a tissue construct and have been designed to provide a sustained local release of cytokines.[6] Scaffolds consisting of natural polymers have recently been developed and have gained popularity. Natural polymers can be considered the first biodegradable biomaterials used in human clinical conditions.[7] These natural materials, due to their bioactive properties, tend to have greater biological interaction with the cells, which allow them to perform better in biological systems. These polymers can be classified as proteins (silk, collagen, fibrinogen, elastin, keratin, actin, and myosin) and polysaccharides (cellulose, amylose, dextran, chitin, and glycosaminoglycans) or polynucleotides (DNA and RNA).[7]

It is often beneficial for scaffolds to mimic the natural ECM because ECM components specifically modulate mesenchymal stem cell (MSC) adhesion, migration, proliferation, and osteogenic differentiation.[8] Cell-derived decellularized ECM is also a promising approach to obtain ECM-based biomimetic material.[9]

When the biomaterial is inserted into a living tissue, a cascade of events is initiated that starts with the adsorption of biomaterials to the material's surface. The immediate interaction of the biomaterial with the in vivo environment is the surface charge and surface energy of the biomaterial. An increase in surface energy improves the wettability of the material surface facilitating the adsorption of serum proteins and other biomolecules, such as fibronectin.[4] This initial wetting (flash spread) that is accompanied by the adsorption of biomolecules is one of the most important preconditions for cells or molecules to become attached to the material surface and to establish tissue contact with the biomaterial. Surface energy and charge depend largely on the material composition and the surface texture. Metals and mineralized materials commonly have a negative surface charge under physiologic conditions due to the presence of oxide molecules on their surface. This results in the adsorption of positively charged molecules to the biomaterial surface. Polymers, such as polylactic acid, have a low surface energy and, therefore, a hydrophobic surface characteristic. The higher surface energy of many metals and ceramics and hydrophilic surfaces can enhance tissue integration. The surface texture of the biomaterial also affects the interaction between itself and the living tissues. Microrough surfaces enhance cellular attachment and differentiation and increased surface roughness increases surface energy and improves wettability.[1]

Another positive effect on cellular behavior is mediated through the microtexture itself as evidenced by surface modification of titanium implants.[4] Different degrees of surface roughness have been shown to modify cellular production of receptors that mediate adhesion to titanium surfaces and increase secretion of osteogenic factors that induce differentiation of cells in contact with the microtextured surface. This leads to the production of cytokines involved in bone formation.[5] Theses finding demonstrate how material science can contribute to the success of tissue engineering by optimizing immediate and late interactions between seeded cells in vitro and living tissue in vivo after implantation. Tissues in the craniomaxillofacial region are varied in composition but essentially consist of a matrix and various cell types. The matrix represents a 3-D structure for cells (scaffolds), which provides them with a specific environment and architecture for a given function.[6]

It is broadly agreed that a scaffold (3-D matrix) should have the following properties: (1) biocompatibility, including degradation products, both of which must not elicit an inflammatory response; (2) noncytotoxicity, including both the material itself and its degradation products, (3) being noncarcinogenic; (4) being sterilizable; (5) predictable physical and mechanical properties, including elasticity, load bearing, and shear stress capacity that are appropriate to the tissue they intend to replace; (6) favorable surgical manipulation properties, including suturing as required for soft tissue implantation and being able to be drilled and hold screws and hardware as required for bone and cartilage scaffolds; (7) porosity with at least an open pore size of 100 μm to 200 μm to allow cellular migration and vascularization and permeation of nutrients, cytokines, and waste; (8) histoconductivity, which guides and stimulates proliferation of autogenous progenitor cells that migrate from surrounding tissues into the scaffold; (9) histoinductivity that induces proliferation and differentiation of autogenous progenitor cells that have migrated from surrounding tissues into the scaffold; and (10) having sites for cellular binding as well as in vivo drug delivery, including growth factors and genes.[4]

VASCULARIZATION AND FABRICATION TECHNIQUES

The vascularization problem associated with larger tissue constructs is complex and has limited the clinical use of prefabricated tissue constructs. Scaffolds should have an interconnected pore structure and high porosity to ensure cellular population and adequate diffusion of nutrients to cells within the construct and to the ECM formed by these cells. Interconnection of the pores is necessary to allow diffusion of waste products from the scaffold because the products of scaffold degradation should be able to exit without interference with other tissues. The mean pore size of the construct is critically important because the cells interact with scaffolds via ligands on the material surface.[7]

Scaffolds with pore sizes larger than 200 μm require a preformed vascular network to supply adequate nutrients, gas exchange, and the removal of waste from the cells within the scaffold.[8] Several different fabrication techniques have been in use to create such scaffolds, including particle leaching, freeze drying, phase separation, fiber mesh formation using melt-spum or solution-spun techniques, electrospinning fiber formation, and solid free-form fabrication.[7–12] The purpose of these different fabrication techniques is to create a scaffold with adequate porosity to accommodate vascular networking used in combination with endothelial progenitor cells. If successful, this technique produces a performed vascular tissue, ex vivo, which can eventually be implanted.[13,14]

Biofabrication of living structures with desired topology and functionality requires an interdisciplinary effort of practitioners of the physical, biological, and engineering sciences. Such efforts are being undertaken in many laboratories around the world. Numerous approaches are pursued, such as those based on the use of natural or artificial scaffolds, decellularized cadaveric extracellular matrices, and bioprinting. To be successful it is crucial to provide in vitro microenvironmental clues for the cells resembling those in the organism. Scaffolds populated with differentiated cells or stem cells of increasing complexity and sophistication are being fabricated. No matter how sophisticated scaffolds are, they can still cause problems stemming from their degradation, eliciting immunogenic reactions and other unforeseen complications. It is now realized that ultimately the best approach might be to rely on the natural self-assembly and self-organizing properties of cells and tissues and the innate regenerative capability of the organism itself. There are different strategies for the fabrication of 3-D biological structures, in particular bioprinting, which uses a biological, scaffoldless, print-based engineering approach that includes self-assembling multicellular units as bioink particles and early developmental morphogenetic principles, such as cell sorting and tissue fusion.[15]

Self-organizing vascular constructs are among the most promising scaffoldless engineered tissues currently in preclinical and clinical studies. Initial successes with in vitro studies on cell sheet engineering of human vascular tissue led to the development of self-organizing vascular constructs.[16]

Self-organization in tissue engineering refers to engineered tissues, which exhibit the generation of distinct structures or gross morphology reminiscent of native tissues without exogenous scaffolds. It is distinct from the self-assembling process in that external manipulation occurs (ie, bioprinting of cells to their appropriate positions and thermal variation to detach a cell sheet).[17]

Application of negative pressure to the gingival tissue has been shown to stimulate neovascularization and enhance tissue repair. Investigators have applied a vacuum suction device to the attached gingival tissue to stimulate local angiogenesis and lymphogenesis. Negative pressure (vacuum/suction) is a mechanical facilitator for vascular network production forming new collateral arterioles and veins along with lymphatic counterparts[18] to respond to local inflammation induced by mechanical irritation.

ADVANCES IN BIOMATERIALS

Chitosan is an interesting biomaterial receiving significant attention in biomaterial research. It is a copolymer made of D-glucosamine and N-acetyl-D-glucosamine bonds and β bonds (1–4) in which glucosamine is the predominant repeating unit in its structure; it is a derivative of the alkaline deacetylation of chitin. It is the second most abundant natural polymer and is found in the shells of crustaceans and walls of fungi.[19,20] Chitosan has been shown to promote wound healing and induce bone formation and also has inhibitory effects on microorganisms. Among the antimicrobial effects of chitosan are those related to *Candida albicans, Enterobacter cloacae, Enterococcus faecalis, Escherichia coli, Klebsiella pneumoniae, Pseudomonas aeruginosa, Staphylococcus aureus,* and *Streptococcus pyogenes.* This inhibitory property is of special significance because it has been proved that the antimicrobial agents, such as bandaging materials and dressings, generally lead to cytotoxicity, delaying the healing process or leading to pathogen resistance. In cases of chitosan, there is almost no need to use an additional dressing because the antimicrobial effects come directly from the membrane. For chitosan scaffolding to be used as structural support in tissue regeneration, it should be highly porous to have the proper cell proliferation at the site of action and have enough surface area for live cells to accommodate adequately, have the correct pore size so that the growing cells can penetrate and proliferate, and have highly interconnected pore structures to allow the transport of nutrients that support cells metabolism and growth.[19–21]

The popularity of chitosan for tissue repair and regeneration stems from the ease of processing and its manufacture in a variety of forms, including fibers, films, sponges, and hydrogels. This processing of Chitosan provides the ability to mimic the shape of the host tissue (biomaterial tissue interface). Moreover, the similarity of its chemical structure to some polysaccharides and ECM constituents offers the possibility of being chemically modified to adapt structurally and functionally to the host tissue.[19]

Atmospheric plasmas are chemically active medias that can be manipulated to generate low or very high temperatures and are referred to as cold or thermal plasmas. Thermal plasma is defined as an ionized gas that has a temperature of several thousand degrees Celsius. It is a high-energy process that strips atoms of their electrons and produces a gas, which flows at a temperature that can exceed 100,000°C. Although plasma is commonly referred to as the fourth state of matter after solids, liquids, and gases, in actuality, hot plasma represents the first state of matter because it makes up 99% of the visible universe in terms of both mass and volume and probably the majority of the invisible universe.[22]

Examples of hot plasma (thermal plasma) include a welding torch, lightning bolt, stars, and the sun. Hot plasma is currently used to sterilize surgical instrument and perform other technical and medical applications.[23]

Atmospheric cold plasma (ACP) was developed initially by NASA and scientists have created cold plasma that functions at 30°C to 40°C and at normal atmospheric pressure. At that temperature, scientists can encounter cold burning plasma flame without injury or burn. Cold plasma technologies are increasingly used in different industries and are used widely in the food industry.

Cold plasmas are able to kill bacteria by damaging microbial DNA and surface structures without being harmful to human tissues. It has been shown that cold plasma is able to kill bacteria growing in biofilms on teeth and in wounds.[22,23]

Antimicrobial properties of cold plasma may usher in a new era in treatment of infections especially in wounds resistant to antibiotic bacteria and biofilms in infected wounds. Studies have demonstrated that ACP was very effective in reducing high concentrations of a planktonic bacterial population to undetectable levels within short treatment times of a few minutes.[24] Additionally, a reduced antimicrobial effect of ACP treatments against bacteria growing in a biofilm form has been reported.[25]

Due to the challenge presented by the persistence of biofilms and lack of techniques to overcome these challenges, an effective control of bacterial biofilms is becoming crucial and should play an important role in the design of disinfection strategies.[26]

Studies have been designed to investigate the potential of ACP for elimination of monoculture biofilms and to examine inhibition potential against bacterial virulence factors and biofilm formation capacity post–ACP treatment. Finally, to examine if ACP-based reduction of virulence factors could further influence the toxicity of *P aeruginosa*, a cytotoxicity assay using CHO-K1 cell line was conducted. The results of this work clearly demonstrated that ACP could be a potential strategy for the inactivation of the established *E coli, Listeria monocytogenes*, and *S aureus* biofilms.[24,25] The type of bacteria, however, in conjunction with its biofilm composition might have an effect on ACP inactivation efficacy. Furthermore, despite the ability of ACP treatment to penetrate and destroy bacterial cells within complex biofilm structures, the bacterial metabolic state and cell morphology could be important factors in determining the inactivation efficacy.

If ACP can be shown to be a predictable agent to destroy bacterial laden biofilm in wounds and on implanted biomaterials, it would represent a tremendous tool to help manage chronic infection associated with implantable devices in the craniomaxillofacial region, such as dental and temporomandibular joint implants.

ACT technology is being studied as a component in skin graft substitutes. Cold plasma has been used for incision closure and skin graft fixation in combination of chitosan film without sutures or staples. The graft biowelding fixation and wound coverage (skin graft) technique enhances healing compared with conventional skin graft technique.[27,28]

The cold plasma product is held in place by Chitoplast strips, which can be positioned alongside the graft/wound edges. In situ chitosan gelation has been reported using ACP as a novel synthetic pathway. This treatment increased the cross-linking density of the chitosan hydrogels and the concentration in the composite. This could be an important pathway for hydrogel synthesis and for polymeric coating on biomaterials.[26]

The combined actions of the dressing and the plasma provide the basis for the normal healing process. The chitosan/ACP film is porous, allowing gas interchange along with wound transexudates. After several days the chitosan is dissolved and the healing occurs. This application eliminates the need for sutures or staples. Cold plasma skin grafts lower the cost for hospitals and reduce infections by enhancing donor site healing.[26]

Chitosan hydrogel applied to skin wounds in diabetic mice enhanced and accelerated wound closure. The chitosan hydrogel combined with fibroblast growth factor type 2 was shown to accelerate the healing process even further. Histology examination showed that this combination fostered the formation of granulation tissue, capillary network, and epithelialization.[27]

Chitosan composites have been successful in bone regeneration in experimental models. Chitosan hydrogel, gelifiable by blue light, was used for bone morphogenetic protein (BMP)-2 release and showed good bone regeneration in a femoral defect in rat.[28] Similar results were observed with the use of a lyophilized porous membrane, a compound of chitosan and hydroxyapatite, in a calvarial defect in the rat. The composite membrane regenerated bone to fill the defect whereas the control site did not and the presence of osteogenic markers was more abundant in the experimental group. Chitosan/nanohydroxyapatite composites are promising regenerative materials because of their ability to induce a robust proliferative response.[28]

Other materials have been synthesized, such as bioactive glass (third-generation) and porous foams, that are designed to activate genes that can stimulate regeneration of living tissues. Efforts are also being made to develop scaffolding materials that possess nanoscale features to mimic the native ECM of the host. Currently a major focus of the researchers is the development of artificial tissues (as biomaterials) that have the architectural features of the natural counterpart.[1]

This new class of biomaterial seems to have a strong osteoinductive capacity, which can be introduced into the scaffolds by surface modification, incorporation of growth factors (eg, transforming growth factor-β, BMP, and vascular endothelial growth factor [VEGF]), seeding bone marrow stem cells. Recent research has shown that BMP-2 and VEGF coloaded into scaffolds enhanced vascularization together with formation of a new bone.[29] Recently gene therapy has been used to modulate osteoinductive properties of growth and transcription factors. Collagen sponge seeded with BMP-9 gene transfected MSCs when implanted in mice have shown promise filling bone defects.[30] Another important factor in bone tissue engineering is modulation of the scaffolds.

Nanophase biomaterial use is an emerging method to produce effective tissue substitutes. The grain size of these materials is in the nanometer range. These materials have shown good osteoclast adhesion, bone remodeling, enhanced osteoblast proliferation, and new bone formation.[23] Nanophase biomaterials have surface and mechanical properties similar to bone so they present with an excellent potential for bone tissue engineering. Their structural dimensions are less than 100 nm.[31] The use of nanomaterials for musculoskeletal tissue repair has 2 advantages. (1) It is a biomimetic approach that mimics the nanodimensional architecture of the native tissue. These materials generate a microenvironment, which signals the infiltrating cells to differentiate and form a neotissue. (2) Mechanical properties of the nanocomposite materials can be tailored to match the native tissue. Successful development of nanobiomaterials in the future may lead to the next generation of musculoskeletal substitute materials; those will be applicable to the biomedical device industry and can improve general health care.[32]

3-D AND 4-D BIOPRINTING

Bioprinting has the potential to be the next step in reconstructive medicine. 3-D bio-printing technologies hold promise for creating biomaterials for use in the craniomaxillofacial region and throughout the body.

3-D printing is the process of producing an object by building it layer by layer. Instead of delivering ink on paper, the printer distributes different materials – ranging from polymers (including plastics) to metal to ceramic – to print an item layer by layer in a process known as additive manufacturing. To create a 3-D object, there is a need for 1 blueprint – a digital file created using modeling software. The computer-generated model is sent to the printer and the selected material is loaded into the device, ready to be heated to allow it to easily flow from the printer nozzle. As it reads the program (blueprint), the printer head moves up and down, side to side, and forward and back, depositing successive layers of chosen materials to build the final product. As each layer is printed, it is transformed into a solid form, either by cooling, chemical reaction (often induced by light), or the mixing of 2 different solutions delivered by the printer head. New layers adhere to previous ones to create a stable, cohesive item. Almost any shape can be created in this way.[33]

Bioprinting works in almost the same way except that instead of delivering materials, such as plastic, ceramics, and metal, it deposits layers of biomaterial that may include living cells to build a complex structure, such as blood vessels or mucosal tissue.[33,34]

The required cells (vascular, mucosal, cartilage, bone, and so forth) are taken from a patient and cultivated until there are enough present to create a bioink, which is loaded into the printer. This is not always possible, so for some tissues, adult stem cells are used and induced to form the described cells. Although it is a complex process requiring detailed designs and models often based on scans

taken directly from a patient, the printer heads deposit the cells exactly when they are needed and an organic object is built using a large number of very thin layers. The bioprinter must also deliver an organic or synthetic glue, such as a dissolvable gel, or collagen scaffold that the cells cannot lock to or grow on. Some cells can assume the correct positioning by themselves.[35]

4-D PRINTING

Shaping is the next development in tissue regeneration. This is also called 4-D printing, where the fourth dimension is time. This emerging technology will allow biomedical scientists to print objects that then reshape themselves or self-assemble over time. These are 3-D printed items that are designed to change shape after they are printed. Examples today include a printed cube that folds before the eyes or a printed pipe able to sense the need to expand or contract. Materials had to be developed that respond to factors other than water, such as heat and light.[33]

SPECIFIC BIOMATERIAL APPLICATIONS
Bone

The engineering of bone tissue constructs is a complex process because bone is vascularized and must be able to withstand extreme mechanical forces, including flexion and torque. Biomaterials used in the manufacturing of bone tissue constructs must have adequate porosity allowing for cellular and vascular in growth, yet excessive porosity weakens the biomaterials and it may not be able to sustain adequate mechanical strength during the incorporation and maintenance phase of bone regeneration.[36] Therefore, the exact balance of porosity and strength has been difficult to attain. Nevertheless, scientists are making progress in this regard and numerous materials and constructs have been investigated.

Bioactive ceramics, in particular calcium phosphate-based ceramics, are able to completely fuse with mineral bone. The mechanical properties of bioactive ceramics can be manipulated by the tissue engineer by varying the ceramic's porosity, creating scaffolds with different fracture toughness, load capacity, and flex tolerance.[37] Bioactive ceramics, however, have lower fracture toughness, load capacities, and flex tolerance compared with natural bone. The drawback of calcium phosphate–based ceramics is that they have long in vivo degradation times, preventing bone remodeling and regeneration. Research into the use of various biodegradable polymers with bioactive ceramics is still needed to create a bone tissue scaffold with mechanical properties similar to those of natural bone.[34] One team of scientists at Swansea University has developed a bioprinting process that can create an artificial bone matrix in the exact shape of the bone request, using a biocompatible material that is strong, durable, and regenerative over a period of 8 to 10 weeks. They then implant the bone construct, which then fuses with and is eventually replaced by the patient's natural bones. The team has been able to print a small bone with architecturally favorable trabecular features in about 2 hours. They envision that they could soon be printed in the operating room while the surgeons work.[38] Another group at the University of Nottingham has used bioprinting to create a bone construct of the bone they are trying to replace. The construct/scaffold is then coated with adult human stem cells capable of developing into the desired tissue type. This is combined with the bioink from the printer, a combination of polylactic acid and alginate, which works as a cushioning material for the cells. The final product is then implanted into the body where the scaffold is resorbed and replaced by new bone. These results are impressive and exciting.[38]

Skin, Mucosa, and Soft Tissue

Bioengineered skin and soft tissue substitutes may be derived from human tissue (autologous or allogenic), nonhuman tissue (xenographic), synthetic material, or a composite of these materials. Bioengineered skin and soft tissue substitutes are being evaluated for a variety of conditions, including burns, avulsion skin injuries, resections for tumors, and intraoral defects. Acellular dermal matrix (ADM) products are also being evaluated in the repair of a variety of soft tissues.[39–41]

Bioengineered skin and soft tissue substitutes may be either acellular or cellular. Acellular products (eg, dermis with cellular material removed) contain a matrix or scaffold composed of materials, such as collagen, hyaluronic acid, and fibronectin. The various ADM products can differ in several ways, including species source (human, bovine, and porcine), tissue source (eg, dermis, pericardium, and intestinal mucosa), additives (eg, antibiotics and surfactants), hydration (wet and freeze dried), and required preparation (multiple rinses and rehydration).[41]

Cellular products contain living cells, such as fibroblasts and keratinocytes, within a matrix. The cell contained within the matrix may be autologous, allogenic, or derived from other species (eg, bovine or porcine). Skin substitutes may also be composed of dermal cells, epidermal cells, or a combination of dermal and epidermal cells and may provide growth factors to stimulate healing. Tissue-engineered skin substitutes can be used as either temporary or permanent wound coverings.[1,42]

There are a large number of potential applications for artificial skin and soft tissue products. One large category is nonhealing wounds, which potentially encompasses diabetic neuropathic ulcers, vascular insufficiency ulcers, and pressure ulcers. A substantial minority of such wounds do not heal adequately with standard wound care, leading to prolong morbidity and increased risk mortality. For example, nonhealing lower-extremity wounds represent an ongoing risk for infection, sepsis, limb amputation, and death. Bioengineered skin and soft tissue substitutes have the potential to improve rates of healing and reduce complications.[43,44]

Other situations in which bioengineered skin products might substitute for living skin grafts include certain postsurgical states, in which skin coverage is inadequate for the procedure performed, or for surgical wounds in patients with a compromised ability to heal. Second-degree and third-degree burns are another situation in which artificial skin products may substitute for autografts or allografts. Certain primary dermatologic conditions that involve large areas of skin breakdown, such as bullous diseases, may also be conditions in which artificial skin products can be considered as substitutes for skin grafts. ADM products are also being evaluated in the repair of other soft tissues, including after oral and facial surgery, and a variety of other conditions.[45]

Skin researchers at Wake Forest School of Medicine have successfully designed a printer that can print skin cells directly onto a burn wound. A scanner determines the size and depth of the wound and this information is passed to the printer. After relevant cells have been cultivated, the printer applies the correct cell types at the correct depth to cover the wound. With this technology the team applies a patch of skin one-tenth the size of the burn to grow enough skin cells for skin printing. Because the 3-D bioprinter prints in layers and because skin is a multilayer organ with different cell types, it is well suited for this type of technology. One company has produced multilayered skin consisting of the dermis and epidermis layers. Some of the challenges that remain include ways to prevent the heat generated by the printer from damaging the cells or their viability. Additionally, the complexities of the tissue include nerves, blood vessels, and other factors that must be considered. The pore sizes recommended for skin scaffolding should be greater than 160 μm, varying between 100 μm and 200 μm, with a desired 90% porosity to provide the necessary space and enough surface to grow cells and create priority temporary scaffolds for implantation, allowing for regeneration or repair of damaged tissue.[8,42] Vascular research engineers in England and the Lawrence Livermore National Laboratory are using bioprinting to create living blood vessels. They have created materials and a microenvironment created by their bioprinters in such a way that enables small blood vessels – human capillaries – to develop on their own. It is a slow process; to assist, tubes of cells and other biomaterials are printed out to help deliver vital nutrients to the surrounding printed environment. Over time, the self-assembled capillaries connect with the bioprinted tubes, thereby beginning to deliver nutrients to the cells on their own – mimicking the way their structure works in the human body. Another method of creating blood vessels was developed by using agarose fiber templates covered with hydrogel. Scientist using aqarose fiber templates covered with hydrogel were able to construct microchanel Networks, which exhibited various architectural features.[46] Bioprinting today is mainly used for simulating and reconstructing hard tissue and for preparing drug-delivery systems. The fabrication of 3-D structures with living cells and bioactive moieties spatially distributed throughout will be a reality in the near future. Fabrication of complex tissues and organs, however, is still at the development stage and is at least 10 years away.[46]

Nerve Tissue Engineering

Peripheral nerve injuries can result from mechanical, thermal, chemical, congenital, or pathologic etiologies. Peripheral nerves possess the capacity of self-regeneration, which represents an important difference from the central nervous system. In cases of loss of neural function of important peripheral nerves, nerve regeneration requires a complex interplay between cells, ECM, growth factors, and the guidance of nerve fibers.[47] The combination of natural or synthetic nerve conduits (filled or open lumen) used as a guidance channel with local growth factor delivery has been demonstrated to show promising results during the past 2 decades.[48] Predictability, however, is still not ideal.

Currently, Food and Drug Administration–approved collagen nerve conduits, such as Neura-Gen and the NeuraWrap (Integra, New Jersey), are used as guidance channels in the treatment of injured peripheral nerves.[49] Due to the important physiologic role of Schwann cells, cell transplantation represents yet another strategy to create the optimal microenvironment for nerve regeneration. Studies using autogenous Schwann cells for their tissue-engineering nerve constructs were able to obtain improved axonal growth.[49,50] Directed neuronal differentiation and single or multiple protein delivery using embryonic or adult stem cells are alternatives to Schwann cell therapy[49,51] but are still in the developmental stages.

Skeletal Muscle Tissue Engineering

The design endpoint of tendon tissue engineering is to create a substitute that is able to withstand forces that are greater than the peak forces seen in vivo.[52] Tendon tissue constructs have been made using MSCs in combination with hydrogel and tissue engineering[53] sponge scaffolds. These scaffolds are composed of polymers and proteins, such as collagen.[54] Advances in ex vivo culture conditions, such as cell culture on a scaffold under tension, have been shown to increase the strength of the tendon tissue constructs both ex vivo and after implantation at 12 weeks.[55,56] Tissue engineers have also found that alteration in the cell to matrix ratio has an effect on the load-bearing capacity of tendon tissue constructs.[57] Unlike smooth muscle, in which muscle contraction is in multiple directions, skeletal muscle requires a tissue construct that produces uniaxial contractions. The cells for such a muscle tissue construct can potentially be derived from satellite progenitor cells found in adult striated muscle or from mesenchymal adult stem cells.[58] The use of an aligned scaffold, such as collagen has been explored with different cell seeding techniques in an attempt to form a tissue construct that has the desired unidirectional orientation.[59] This has proved a difficult problem, and further research involving cell implantation techniques and scaffold construction is required.

Complex Oral Tissue Regeneration

Transplantation of bioengineered tooth germs into the oral environment has been attempted to produce a whole tooth. The use of biodegradable polyglycolic/polylactide scaffolds shaped like a tooth and seeded with cells isolated from postnatal porcine third molar tooth buds were transplanted into rats for 20 to 30 weeks and successfully produced recognizable tooth structures.[60] however, the size of the bioengineered tooth did not conform to the shape and size of the natural tooth.[61]

Regeneration technologies for complex oral tissue/organs, such as teeth, salivary glands, mandibular condyle, and tongue, have not yet reached the clinical trial stage because of their developmental and structural complexity.

Recent advances in animal research have identified feasible strategies to regenerate these tissues. Regeneration of the tooth root, however, is currently a more realistic and clinically applicable approach, because the regenerated root can be used as an abutment for a fixed prosthesis (new stem cell–based technology for regeneration).[4,12]

Mandibular Condyle Regeneration

The combination of cartilage tissue progenitor cells carried on a hydrogel scaffold and distraction osteogenesis has been successfully used to reconstruct a condylar defect in a goat model. A human-shaped condyle was successfully engineered from chondrogenetic and osteogenetic rat bone marrow stem cells, encapsulated in a biocompatible polymer. These findings may provide a proof of concept for ultimate stem cell–based tissue engineering of degenerated articular condyle diseases, such as arthritis.[4,62]

Tongue Regeneration

Cell-based reconstruction of the tongue was reported in a rat model where myoblast/progenitor cells carried in a collagen gel were implanted into the hemiglossectomized tongue to provide successful muscle regeneration in the tongue with reduced scar contracture. The application of cyclic strain to bone marrow–derived stem cells greatly accelerated in vitro skeletal biogenesis to achieve a lined myotube structure seemingly necessary for creating a physiologically relevant environment to engineer skeletal muscle.[62]

THE FUTURE OF BIOMATERIALS AND TISSUE ENGINEERING

The irrational exuberance of the scientific community associated with the emergence of stem cell therapy and tissue engineering has been tempered by the realization that the process of regenerative medicine is more complex and difficult to achieve than initially expected. Further basic science research in the fields of material sciences, gene therapy, and cell and developmental biology will provide better insight into the overall potential of tissue engineering and the problems it currently faces. Eventually, scientific advances in tissue engineering and biomaterials will allow for better tissue constructs that will improve the overall success rates in reconstructive surgery using regenerative medicine techniques. The best source of stem cells for the tissue engineer has yet to be determined: either autogenesis versus allogeneic cells or embryonic versus adult stem cells. Evolving ethical and political considerations play a role in the future research of stem cells and their applications in regenerative medicine. The use of adult stem cells is attractive, because it avoids the potential ethical and political milieu that surrounds the use of embryonic stem cells.[61] Both the autogenous adult stem cell and the allogeneic embryonic stem cell using will likely require time for the manufacturing of tissue constructs and are unlikely to be used in acute fashion. Research with tissue-engineered skin substitutes will likely involve the refinement of products that manipulate growth factors, allowing for a more rapid healing of wounds. Advancements will also likely involve the combination of skin tissue constructs with deep soft tissue constructs, such as subcutaneous tissue and fascia. Ongoing research is attempting to identify sources of cells capable of producing articular cartilage or creating a tissue that simulates articular cartilages' hydrostatic pressures and ability to withstand dynamic compression forces. The development of a zonal cartilage tissue construct will play an important role in the development of future tissue-engineered cartilage substitutes. Advancements in tissue engineering of bone will likely result in tissue constructs that are composed of biodegradable polymers combined with either bioactive glasses or ceramics. This would create a product with load capacities and fracture toughness similar to those of natural bone. Bone tissue constructs will likely expand to include the use of growth factor and cytokines to increase the rate at which fracture repair and regeneration occur. In the future, more complex devices (nerve conduits, delivery systems, bioengineered nerve grafts, and so forth) will be needed. A better understanding of the complexity of growth factor therapy and genetic engineering may help find better solutions to restore functional peripheral nerve tissue. If a solution to the vascularization issue with complex tissues and organs is found, it will have broad applications to fields of tissue engineering and bioartificial organ construction.

REFERENCES

1. Bhat S, Kumar A. Biomaterials and bioengineering tomorrow's healthcare. Biomatter 2013;3.
2. Fassina L, Saino E, Visai L, et al. Electromagnetic stimulation to optimize the bone regeneration capacity of gelatin-based cryogels. Int J Immunopathol Pharmacol 2012;25:165–74.
3. Anderson JM. The future of biomedical materials. J Mater Sci Mater Med 2006;17:1025–8.
4. Abou Neel EA, Chrzanowski W, Salih VM, et al. Tissue engineering in dentistry. J Dent 2014;42:915–28.

5. Boyan BD, Batzer R, Kieswetter K, et al. Titanium surface roughness alters responsiveness of MG63 osteoblast-like cells to 1 alpha,25-(OH)2D3. J Biomed Mater Res 1998;39:77–85.

6. Kieswetter K, Schwartz Z, Hummert TW, et al. Surface roughness modulates the local production of growth factors and cytokines by osteoblast-like MG-63 cells. J Biomed Mater Res 1996;32:55–63.

7. Loh QL, Choong C. Three-dimensional scaffolds for tissue engineering applications: role of porosity and pore size. Tissue Eng Part B Rev 2013;19:485–502.

8. Melek LN. Tissue engineering in oral and maxillofacial reconstruction. Tanta Dental J 2015;12:211–23.

9. Gomes ME, Ribeiro AS, Malafaya PB, et al. A new approach based on injection moulding to produce biodegradable starch-based polymeric scaffolds: morphology, mechanical and degradation behaviour. Biomaterials 2001;22:883–9.

10. Hottot A, Vessot S, Andrieu J. Determination of mass and heat transfer parameters during freeze-drying cycles of pharmaceutical products. PDA J Pharm Sci Technol 2005;59:138–53.

11. Wu GH, Hsu S. Review: polymeric-based 3D printing for tissue engineering. J Med Biol Eng 2015;35:285–92.

12. Jia H, Zhu G, Vugrinovich B, et al. Enzyme-carrying polymeric nanofibers prepared via electrospinning for use as unique biocatalysts. Biotechnol Prog 2002;18:1027–32.

13. Amini AR, Laurencin CT, Nukavarapu SP. Bone Tissue Engineering: Recent Advances and Challenges. Crit Rev Biomed Eng 2012;40:363–408.

14. Hasan A, Paul A, Vrana NE, et al. Microfluidic techniques for development of 3D vascularized tissue. Biomaterials 2014;35:7308–25.

15. Jakab K, Norotte C, Marga F, et al. Tissue engineering by self-assembly and bio-printing of living cells. Biofabrication 2010;2:022001.

16. Peck M, Gebhart D, Dusserre N, et al. The evolution of vascular tissue engineering and current state of the art. Cells Tissues Organs 2012;195:144–58.

17. Groschel AH, Walther A, Lobling TI, et al. Guided hierarchical co-assembly of soft patchy nanoparticles. Nature 2013;503:247–51.

18. Budinskaya OV, Kontogiorgos ED, Brownlee M, et al. Vacuum-induced suction stimulates increased numbers of blood vessels in healthy dog gingiva. Wounds 2012;24:99–109.

19. Akman AC, Seda Tığlı R, Gümüşderelioğlu M, et al. Bone morphogenetic protein-6-loaded chitosan scaffolds enhance the osteoblastic characteristics of MC3T3-E1 cells. Artif Organs 2010;34:65–74.

20. Rodríguez-Vázquez M, Vega-Ruiz B, Ramos-Zúñiga R, et al. Chitosan and its potential use as a scaffold for tissue engineering in regenerative medicine. Biomed Res Int 2015;2015:821279.

21. Wu H-D, Ji D-Y, Chang W-J, et al. Chitosan-based polyelectrolyte complex scaffolds with antibacterial properties for treating dental bone defects. Mater Sci Eng C 2012;32:207–14.

22. Ermolaeva SA, Varfolomeev AF, Chernukha MY, et al. Bactericidal effects of non-thermal argon plasma in vitro, in biofilms and in the animal model of infected wounds. J Med Microbiol 2011;60:75–83.

23. Ziuzina D, Patil S, Cullen P, et al. Atmospheric cold plasma inactivation of Escherichia coli in liquid media inside a sealed package. J Appl Microbiol 2013;114:778–87.

24. Ziuzina D, Boehm D, Patil S, et al. Cold plasma inactivation of bacterial biofilms and reduction of quorum sensing regulated virulence factors. PLoS One 2015;10:e0138209.

25. Kvam E, Davis B, Mondello F, et al. Nonthermal atmospheric plasma rapidly disinfects multidrug-resistant microbes by inducing cell surface damage. Antimicrob Agents Chemother 2012;56:2028–36.

26. Hants Y, Kabiri D, Drukker L, et al. Preliminary evaluation of novel skin closure of Pfannenstiel incisions using cold helium plasma and chitosan films. J Matern Fetal Neonatal Med 2014;27:1637–42.

27. Ikeda T, Ikeda K, Yamamoto K, et al. Fabrication and characteristics of chitosan sponge as a tissue engineering scaffold. Biomed Res Int 2014;2014:8.

28. Kim S, Bedigrew K, Guda T, et al. Novel osteoinductive photo-cross-linkable chitosan-lactide-fibrinogen hydrogels enhance bone regeneration in critical size segmental bone defects. Acta Biomater 2014;10:5021–33.

29. Kempen DH, Lu L, Heijink A, et al. Effect of local sequential VEGF and BMP-2 delivery on ectopic and orthotopic bone regeneration. Biomaterials 2009;30:2816–25.

30. Kimelman-Bleich N, Pelled G, Zilberman Y, et al. Targeted gene-and-host progenitor cell therapy for nonunion bone fracture repair. Mol Ther 2011;19:53–9.

31. Christenson EM, Anseth KS, van den Beucken JJ, et al. Nanobiomaterial applications in orthopedics. J Orthop Res 2007;25:11–22.

32. Egli RJ, Luginbuehl R. Tissue engineering - nanomaterials in the musculoskeletal system. Swiss Med Wkly 2012;142:w13647.

33. Zhang YS, Yue K, Aleman J, et al. 3D bioprinting for tissue and organ fabrication. Ann Biomed Eng 2016. [Epub ahead of print].

34. Murphy SV, Atala A. 3D bioprinting of tissues and organs. Nat Biotechnol 2014;32:773–85.

35. Pati F, Ha D-H, Jang J, et al. Biomimetic 3D tissue printing for soft tissue regeneration. Biomaterials 2015;62:164–75.

36. Rezwan K, Chen QZ, Blaker JJ, et al. Biodegradable and bioactive porous polymer/inorganic composite scaffolds for bone tissue engineering. Biomaterials 2006;27:3413–31.

37. Brown S, Clarke I, Williams P (Key Engineering Materials, Vol. 218–220). Bioceramics 14, Proceedings of the 14th International Symposium on Ceramics in Medicine. Palm Springs (CA), 14-17th November, 2001.

38. Zelen CM, Serena TE, Denoziere G, et al. A prospective randomised comparative parallel study of amniotic membrane wound graft in the management of diabetic foot ulcers. Int Wound J 2013;10:502–7.

39. A ba-bai-ke-re MM, Wen H, Huang HG, et al. Randomized controlled trial of minimally invasive surgery using acellular dermal matrix for complex anorectal fistula. World J Gastroenterol 2010;16: 3279–86.

40. Fleshman JW, Beck DE, Hyman N, et al. A prospective, multicenter, randomized, controlled study of non-cross-linked porcine acellular dermal matrix fascial sublay for parastomal reinforcement in patients undergoing surgery for permanent abdominal wall ostomies. Dis Colon Rectum 2014;57:623–31.

41. Reyzelman A, Crews RT, Moore JC, et al. Clinical effectiveness of an acellular dermal regenerative tissue matrix compared to standard wound management in healing diabetic foot ulcers: a prospective, randomised, multicentre study. Int Wound J 2009;6:196–208.

42. Falanga V, Margolis D, Alvarez O, et al. Rapid healing of venous ulcers and lack of clinical rejection with an allogeneic cultured human skin equivalent. Human Skin Equivalent Investigators Group. Arch Dermatol 1998;134:293–300.

43. Brigido SA, Boc SF, Lopez RC. Effective management of major lower extremity wounds using an acellular regenerative tissue matrix: a pilot study. Orthopedics 2004;27:s145–149.

44. Kavros SJ, Dutra T, Gonzalez-Cruz R, et al. The use of PriMatrix, a fetal bovine acellular dermal matrix, in healing chronic diabetic foot ulcers: a prospective multicenter study. Adv Skin Wound Care 2014;27: 356–62.

45. Lazic T, Falanga V. Bioengineered skin constructs and their use in wound healing. Plast Reconstr Surg 2011;127(Suppl 1):75S–90S.

46. Murphy SV, Atala A. 3D boprinting of tissue and organs nature Biotechnology 2014;32:773–85. Available at: http://www.nova.org.au/people-medicine/bioprinting.

47. Pfister LA, Papaloizos M, Merkle HP, et al. Nerve conduits and growth factor delivery in peripheral nerve repair. J Peripher Nerv Syst 2007;12:65–82.

48. Archibald SJ, Krarup C, Shefner J, et al. A collagen-based nerve guide conduit for peripheral nerve repair: an electrophysiological study of nerve regeneration in rodents and nonhuman primates. J Comp Neurol 1991;306:685–96.

49. Evans GR, Brandt K, Katz S, et al. Bioactive poly(L-lactic acid) conduits seeded with Schwann cells for peripheral nerve regeneration. Biomaterials 2002; 23:841–8.

50. Whitworth IH, Brown RA, Dore C, et al. Orientated mats of fibronectin as a conduit material for use in peripheral nerve repair. J Hand Surg Br 1995;20: 429–36.

51. Mimura T, Dezawa M, Kanno H, et al. Peripheral nerve regeneration by transplantation of bone marrow stromal cell-derived Schwann cells in adult rats. J Neurosurg 2004;101:806–12.

52. Shearn JT, Juncosa-Melvin N, Boivin GP, et al. Mechanical stimulation of tendon tissue engineered constructs: effects on construct stiffness, repair biomechanics, and their correlation. J Biomech Eng 2007;129:848–54.

53. Vaz CM, Fossen M, van Tuil RF, et al. Casein and soybean protein-based thermoplastics and composites as alternative biodegradable polymers for biomedical applications. J Biomed Mater Res A 2003;65:60–70.

54. Caplan AI. Review: mesenchymal stem cells: cell-based reconstructive therapy in orthopedics. Tissue Eng 2005;11:1198–211.

55. Awad HA, Butler DL, Boivin GP, et al. Autologous mesenchymal stem cell-mediated repair of tendon. Tissue Eng 1999;5:267–77.

56. Juncosa-Melvin N, Matlin KS, Holdcraft RW, et al. Mechanical stimulation increases collagen type I and collagen type III gene expression of stem cell-collagen sponge constructs for patellar tendon repair. Tissue Eng 2007;13:1219–26.

57. Awad HA, Butler DL, Harris MT, et al. In vitro characterization of mesenchymal stem cell-seeded collagen scaffolds for tendon repair: effects of initial seeding density on contraction kinetics. J Biomed Mater Res 2000;51:233–40.

58. Yost MJ, Simpson D, Wrona K, et al. Design and construction of a uniaxial cell stretcher. Am J Physiol Heart Circ Physiol 2000;279:H3124–30.

59. Yan W, George S, Fotadar U, et al. Tissue engineering of skeletal muscle. Tissue Eng 2007;13:2781–90.

60. Ikeda E, Morita R, Nakao K, et al. Fully functional bioengineered tooth replacement as an organ replacement therapy. Proc Natl Acad Sci U S A 2009;106:13475–80.

61. Young CS, Terada S, Vacanti JP, et al. Tissue engineering of complex tooth structures on biodegradable polymer scaffolds. J Dent Res 2002;81: 695–700.

62. Egusa H, Sonoyama W, Nishimura M, et al. Stem cells in dentistry–Part II: Clinical applications. J Prosthodont Res 2012;56:229–48.

Index

Oral Maxillofacial Surg Clin N Am 29 (2017) 117–120
http://dx.doi.org/10.1016/S1042-3699(16)30124-8
1042-3699/17

Moving?

Make sure your subscription moves with you!

To notify us of your new address, find your **Clinics Account Number** (located on your mailing label above your name), and contact customer service at:

Email: journalscustomerservice-usa@elsevier.com

800-654-2452 (subscribers in the U.S. & Canada)
314-447-8871 (subscribers outside of the U.S. & Canada)

Fax number: 314-447-8029

Elsevier Health Sciences Division
Subscription Customer Service
3251 Riverport Lane
Maryland Heights, MO 63043

*To ensure uninterrupted delivery of your subscription, please notify us at least 4 weeks in advance of move.

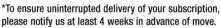

Printed and bound by CPI Group (UK) Ltd, Croydon, CR0 4YY

08/05/2025

01864696-0010